HV 2504.5 .U6 C73 1987
Crammatte, Alan B.
Meeting the challenge

R0069I 96583   24.95

THE CHICAGO PUBLIC LIBRARY
CONRAD SULZER REGIONAL LIBRARY
4455 LINCOLN AVE.
CHICAGO, ILLINOIS 60625

FORM 19

SEP   1989

MEETING THE
CHALLENGE

MEETING THE CHALLENGE

Hearing-Impaired Professionals in the Workplace

Alan B. Crammatte

With Chapters by
Terry H. Coye
Steven L. Jamison
John G. Schroedel

Gallaudet University Press
Washington, D.C.

Gallaudet University Press, Washington, DC 20002
© 1987 by Gallaudet University. All rights reserved
Published 1987
Printed in the United States of America

Library of Congress Cataloging in Publication Data

Crammatte, Alan B.
  Meeting the challenge.

  Bibliography: p.
  Includes index.
  1. Deaf—Employment—United States—Longitudinal studies. 2. Hearing impaired—Employment—United States—Longitudinal studies. 3. Professional employees—United States—Longitudinal studies.
  I. Title.
  HV2504.5.U6C73   1987   331.5′9   87-118
  ISBN 0-930323-24-6

Gallaudet University is an equal opportunity employer/educational institution. Programs and services offered by Gallaudet University receive substantial financial support from the U.S. Department of Education.

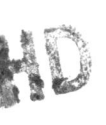

To Florence, right hand in all of my endeavors

Contents

Preface　　　ix
Prologue　　A Humanitarian Era　*1*
Chapter One　　The Professional Environment　*13*
Chapter Two　　Communication　*25*
Chapter Three　Education　*35*
Chapter Four　Job Finding Methods, *Terry H. Coye*　*47*
Chapter Five　Working Conditions　*73*
Chapter Six　Predictors of Socioeconomic Status, *John G. Schroedel*　*93*
Chapter Seven　Comparing the Eras　*139*
Chapter Eight　Perspectives on Employment, *Steven L. Jamison*　*167*
Chapter Nine　Summary and Conclusions　*177*

Appendix A　The Problem and the Approach　*183*
Appendix B　Describing Hearing Impairment　*191*
Appendix C　Professional Employment Questionnaire　*195*
Appendix D　Distribution of Occupations—All Respondents　*205*
Appendix E　Distribution of Occupations—1982 Comparison Group　*209*
Appendix F　Indexes of Job Satisfaction and Rejection　*213*
Reference List　*215*
Index　*229*

Preface

In 1960 a study was made of deaf people in professional occupations. It revealed that, despite the negative stereotyped views of the general public, a few deaf persons had succeeded in obtaining professional positions in offices and laboratories where speech was the normal mode of communication.

During the 1960s and 1970s the United States experienced a quantum leap in awareness and legislation regarding people with disabilities. Hearing-impaired people have benefited from this humanitarian wave and their own more assertive public image. The benefits have included greatly expanded opportunities for postsecondary education, active interest and recruitment by some employers, and, in general, greater public interest and knowledge about deaf people and their capabilities. (The Prologue contains a more detailed examination of these developments.)

In 1982, therefore, it seemed appropriate to attempt another study of deaf professional workers. The objective of the new study was to determine how well deaf persons had responded to the increase in public awareness and the new opportunities created by that awareness. The chance to conduct such a study came with my appointment to the Powrie Doctor Chair of Deaf Studies at Gallaudet College in 1982.

The 1982 study was more inclusive than the 1960 study. The later study used a mail survey rather than direct interviews as the information-gathering technique. A complete description of the methodology is presented in Appendix A.

Some people who serve hearing-impaired clients use the term *"hearing-impaired"* to describe people whose hearing is usable to some degree. This definition distinguishes *hearing-impaired* people from people who are *deaf*. This book uses *hearing-impaired* in the broadest sense to mean any and all degrees of hearing disability. Extent of hearing impairment and other esoteric terms are defined more fully in Appendix B. One other note on terminology—Gallaudet College officially became Gallaudet University in October 1986. Because all of the data presented in this book had been collected and analyzed before this time, all references in the book are to Gallaudet College.

Many people contributed to making this project a reality. John G. Schroedel, a research associate at the Arkansas Rehabilitation Research and Training Center on Deafness and Hearing Impairment, took a very active role in the planning and development of the 1982 survey. His broad background in the field of employment of hearing-impaired persons lent important perspective to the study. In addition, he also wrote chapter 6, which examines the socioeconomic attainments of this group. Terry H. Coye, professor of English at Gallaudet University, performed a separate study of job-finding methods using a sample of the population of this study. His results are found in chapter 4. Steven L. Jamison, a distinguished personnel consultant with IBM and an active promoter of employment for people with hearing disabilities, offers his observations on employer attitudes toward hearing-impaired workers in chapter 8. All three contributors also reviewed the entire manuscript.

David Armstrong, Donald Moores, and Ronald Sutcliffe, all of Gallaudet University (as are all of the contributors mentioned below), served with Dr. Schroedel on the oversight committee. Robert C. Harmon of the English Department read the manuscript for grammatical fluency.

Technical assistance came from a number of people, including Susan King, who developed the analytical program; James Haynes, who prepared the mailing list program; and John Woo, who assisted in computer techniques.

Members of the deaf community were very cooperative in the initial canvass. They provided names and addresses of hearing-impaired acquaintances deemed to be in professional employment. The respondents, themselves, recognized the potential value of the study and responded to the questionnaire fully and promptly. Many provided names and addresses of other potential respondents.

The following student aides did much of the computer input and verification: J. Wellington Fahnebulleh, III, Dora Giraldo, Sally Lee, and Norma Jean Taylor. The manuscript was processed under the direction of Robert Johnson, assisted by Dotti Smith. Editing for publication was done by Ivey Pittle of Gallaudet University Press.

Prologue
A HUMANITARIAN ERA

The main aim in proposing this study was to compare deaf professional workers and their working conditions in 1960 and 1982. Comparisons of such widely spaced years are really meaningful only if the period between has been one of sufficient change to make the two years significantly different. The era 1960–1982 certainly meets the criterion of change as regards social and economic conditions for hearing-impaired Americans. These years saw a humanitarian revolution that brought many hearing-impaired citizens out of the closet of meek isolation into the active arena of competition for training, jobs, and recognition.

Detailing the progress made in the community of hearing-impaired people would require a book in itself. While this would be an appealing and worthwhile tome, that much depth and breadth is not required in the present study. Instead, this chapter presents, in timeline-form, a text explaining very briefly each change and its importance for the hearing-impaired community. The following timeline lists the important events that occurred during this period. The text that follows covers only the period 1960 to 1980; however, a few events preceding that period are shown because they were seminal causes of progress. The citations represent early references in print to the events chronicled.

Timeline
The Dynamic Years: 1960–1980

1960　Ft. Monroe #1; Jr. NAD

1961　Ft. Monroe #2; LTP, CSUN; Riverside CC; PL 86-276

1963　Continuing education, CSUN

1964　NAD; RID; Centennial Fund, GC; Acoustic coupler; ODAS; IPO

1965　Dictionary of ASL; Babbidge report; Captioned films expands

1966　MSSD; DRTC, NYU; PRWAD (ADARA); NAD Executive Secretary

1967　COSD; NTD, first tour; Communication Skills Program; BEH; IAPD

1968　TC public school program; TDI; Delgado CC; Bell and Gallaudet scholarships

1969　NTID

1970　PL 91-587

1971　Captioned TV; Deaf actors on Broadway and on television

1972　Deaf Awareness Week

1973　Halex House; Vocational Rehabilitation Act of 1973

1974　NCDP; EPOC

1975　PL 94-142; NCLD; Regional Employment Seminars

1976　LDF; NAD

1978　Special School of the Future; TC grows; NCED

1980　SWCID

1944: *Gallaudet College* (enrollment 145 at the time) began plans for expansion after agitation by alumni and a federal study. Much better professional preparation resulted from this growth (Gallagher, 1949).

1945: *The Office of Vocational Rehabilitation (OVR)* appointed Boyce R. Williams to its staff. Williams was the first deaf person to fill a federal position involving deafness. His influence in the councils of the federal government relative to hearing impairment far exceeded the bounds of his job ("Deaf Man Chosen," 1945).

1955: *The New York State Psychiatric Institute*, begun on an OVR grant, was the forerunner of numerous mental health services developed for hearing-impaired people during the progressive years (Rainer, Altshuler, & Kallman, 1963).

1958: *Captioned Films for the Deaf*, a service agency that captioned and distributed feature films, was created by Public Law 85–905.

1960: *Fort Monroe Workshop #1*, an OVR-sponsored conference on research, involved mainly hearing school administrators (an ancient paternalistic pattern). However, the two deaf participants so impressed OVR officials that plans began soon after for a gathering of hearing-impaired leaders the next year (Crammatte, 1965).

The Junior National Association of the Deaf was created by the National Association of the Deaf (NAD) to give young people the experience and confidence to become leaders and advocates (Gannon, 1981).

1961: *Fort Monroe Workshop #2* brought local and national deaf leaders and hearing professionals from across the nation to develop organizations and programs that would meet the needs of hearing-impaired people. The workshop was sponsored by the OVR but was administered by deaf persons; it proved to be a watershed for hearing-impaired people. Many of the recommended actions became actualities in subsequent years. More importantly, a ferment grew among deaf leaders which led many a printer and craftsperson to aspire to more challenging roles as full-time professionals or administrators (Crammatte & Schreiber, 1961).

The Leadership Training Program in the Area of Deafness (LTP at California State University, Northridge [CSUN]) was established to train personnel for leadership roles in organizations serving deaf people. The LTP program has accepted people with and without hearing impairments. The LTP has been a powerful factor in awakening hearing-impaired people to their potential for leadership. The program graduates serve today in education, rehabilitation, social services, and organizations of hearing-impaired people (Falberg, 1967).

Riverside Community College was the first college to adapt its course offerings to meet the needs of hearing-impaired students through special support services. This idea did not spread to other colleges until 1968, but currently there are 106 such programs in the United States and Canada (Rawlings, Karchmer, & DeCaro, 1983).

Public Law 87–276 provided funds for programs training teachers to work with hearing- and speech-impaired children. Many programs were expanded or established due to this legislation (Nazzaro, 1977).

1963: *CSUN* initiated the first professionally organized continuing education program. The class began as an experiment of the LTP class. The program created some excitement locally; as time passed, this activity spread nationwide (Henderson, 1964).

1964: *The National Association of the Deaf* moved its headquarters to Washington, D.C. For the previous 18 years, the NAD had been run from the president's den. Once the move was made to

Washington, a new administration took over. Improved opportunities for advocacy and lobbying were soon to be realized (Shaposka, 1972).

The Registry of Interpreters for the Deaf (RID) brought professionalism and ethics to the field of interpreting for persons with hearing difficulties. The resulting spread of this service has enabled hearing-impaired people to participate in activities ranging from PTA meetings to legislative hearings (Youngs, 1967).

The Gallaudet College Centennial Fund divided about $500,000 among three endowments: an alumni house, a cultural fund, and a graduate fellowship fund. Since awarding its first grant in 1968, the fellowship fund has given more than $200,000 to hearing-impaired doctoral candidates (Crammatte, 1982).

Robert Weitbrecht, a deaf physicist, invented the *acoustic coupler*, a device which permits a telephone to be connected to a telecommunications device for the deaf (TDD). The invention has vastly increased telephone communication among hearing-impaired people. As business firms, professional services, and government agencies have installed TDDs, accessibility among hearing-impaired telephone users has grown (Gannon, 1981).

The Oral Deaf Adults Section (ODAS) of the A. G. Bell Association for the Deaf (AGBAD), was established in April. ODAS has provided an organized voice for those hearing-impaired people who were orally taught. The organization has been active in promoting professional employment for hearing-impaired adults ("Oral Deaf Adults," 1964).

The International Parents Organization (IPO), a section of AGBAD, adopted a new name and constitution. Its chief concern has been with education and promotion of better opportunities for hearing-impaired children and adults.

1965: *The Dictionary of American Sign Language on Linguistic Principles*, by William Stokoe, carefully analyzed American Sign Language and concluded that it is, indeed, a true language with its own visual grammatical structure. This information led to greater scholarly interest in sign language and deafness, and it gave hearing-impaired people a renewed sense of pride in their language and a stronger sense of community (Stokoe, 1965).

The Babbidge Report, mandated by Congress in response to questions raised by Gallaudet College alumni, called for more federal aid for teacher training and a reexamination of the existing educational system for hearing-impaired students (Advisory Committee on the Education of the Deaf, 1965).

Captioned Films for the Deaf, established in 1957, was expanded to include educational media. Captioned Films also began conducting research and providing training for teachers who used such educational media (Kundert, 1969).

1966: *The Model Secondary School for the Deaf (MSSD)*, became the first and only regional high school for hearing-impaired students (Nazzaro, 1977). Its innovative teaching aids and services have influenced education of teenagers and hence, indirectly, professional preparation among hearing-impaired persons (Gallaudet College, 1976).

The Deafness Research and Training Center at New York University began serving as a graduate training center for a number of deaf professionals. The center's funding came from the Rehabilitation Services Administration (Norris, 1972).

Professional Rehabilitation Workers with the Adult Deaf (now American Deafness and Rehabilitation Association) was the first professional society for rehabilitation workers serving deaf clients. It has expanded to include all professionals working with deafness (Lauritsen, 1969).

An executive secretary was appointed by the NAD to meet the expanding demands of the Washington, D.C. office. The small, two-person staff has since grown to a large enterprise that occupies its own office building and conducts an extensive publishing program (Shaposka, 1972).

1967: *The Council of Organizations Serving the Deaf (COSD)* was established to provide a single voice for the many groups interested in the welfare of hearing-impaired people. Its daily services and annual forums spotlighted a number of problems and proposed a number of solutions. Unfortuately, it lasted only 5 years (Meek, 1968).

The National Theatre of the Deaf (NTD) made its first tour. The group has played an important public relations role by increasing public awareness of the abilities of deaf people. The NTD has toured the world and won numerous professional awards (Powers, 1969).

The Communication Skills Program of the NAD began promoting the study and teaching of American Sign Language. The program created an increase in the number of sign language classes across the nation that surprised officials and brought sign language out of the closet (Gannon, 1981).

The Bureau of Education of the Handicapped was established in the U.S. Office of Education. This bureau oversees the Captioned Films for the Deaf program. It also funds research, demonstration programs, and scholarships for educators of hearing-impaired children (Adler, 1969).

The International Association of Parents of the Deaf (IAPD) began as a section of the Convention of American Instructors of the Deaf. It later became an independent organization and changed its name to the American Society for Deaf Children. The group has served as an information center for parents and an advocate for better education and social services for hearing-impaired people (Katz, n.d.).

1968: *Total Communication (TC)* was the name given to an educational philosophy that imbued a program for hearing-impaired students in the Santa Ana (California) School District. The phrase encompassed the idea of early communication intervention and subsequent education by all possible means—oral, manual, residual hearing, and other visual stimuli. The philosophy was widely adopted in many schools for deaf children. It also led to an increase in preschool programs and encouraged interaction between hearing and hearing-impaired children in public schools (Jordan, Gustason, & Rosen, 1974).

Telecommunications for the Deaf, Inc. (TDI), was established to promote the use of telecommunication devices among and for hearing-impaired people. TDI has produced an annual national telephone directory. It also has performed a variety of services to TDD users and sales agents and has explored new communication media, such as computer networks and television captioning (Strassler, 1982).

Delgado Community College was established with federal grants to provide a model program for community colleges interested in serving hearing-impaired students. The following year similar demonstration programs were set up at Seattle Community College and St. Paul Technical/Vocational Institute (Rawlings, Karchmer, & DeCaro, 1983; Wells, 1969).

Bell scholarships were first awarded by the AGBAD to orally educated students. Coincidentally, the first awards of the Graduate Fellowship Fund (which was created in 1964 from the Gallaudet College Centennial Fund) were made in this same year. Both programs have aided students seeking professional training ("Bell Scholarship Granted," 1968).

1969: *The National Technical Institute for the Deaf (NTID)* was established at the Rochester Institute of Technology. The program was designed to train hearing-impaired students in technical fields. NTID offers an alternative to the liberal arts program available at Gallaudet College (Frisina, 1971).

1970: *Public Law 91–587* authorized the Kendall School to operate as a demonstration elementary school. This act established demonstration programs ranging from elementary through secondary level on the Gallaudet College campus (Nazzaro, 1971).

1971: *Captioned TV* began at WGBH in Boston in October. That same year the Department of Health, Education, and Welfare began investigating the feasibility of closed captioning television broadcasts (Califano, 1979). Currently, many prime-time programs and commercials are closed captioned. Videocassette makers also have closed captioned many films (Gannon, 1981).

Deaf actors, thanks to exposure via NTD, have appeared in stage and television productions and in their own local companies. A few deaf actors have had continuing roles in regular programs, while others have appeared as guest performers. Some individuals and programs have won awards. This is an entirely new field of employment for hearing-impaired workers, although local amateur performances have a long history (Gannon, 1981).

1972: *Colorado became the first state to officially proclaim a Deaf Awareness Week*. It symbolized increasing awareness by the general public and increasing pride among hearing-impaired people (Gannon, 1981).

1973: *Halex House*, a three-story office building, was purchased by the NAD only 9 years after installing a full-time administrator. Halex House presently contains the NAD offices and the offices of several national organizations related to deafness (*Deaf American*, 1973).

The Vocational Rehabilitation Act of 1973 established forceful regulations for ensuring the civil rights of handicapped people. Section 501 called for affirmative action in the employment of handicapped workers by federal agencies; Section 502 prohibited physical barriers in public accommodations; Section 503 required affirmative action by firms holding federal procurement contracts or grants; and Section 504 banned discrimination under any program receiving federal funds (United States Senate, 1973).

1974: *A national census of the deaf population* was taken to count the hearing-impaired population of the United States. This was the first such attempt since 1930, when the Census Bureau tried but gave up in despair. The Deafness Research and Training Center at NYU prepared the survey under the auspices of the NAD. The census findings have been widely used for everything from program planning to advocacy (Schein & Delk, 1974).

Experiential Programs Off Campus (EPOC) began at Gallaudet College staffed by a single officer. EPOC then served eight students, several federal agencies, and the IBM Corp. By 1982 it was serving 150–200 students a year, placing them in a variety of internships and jobs with private firms, social service agencies, federal agencies, and even some foreign companies. Since EPOC's founding, student employment horizons have been expanded remarkably (Walter, 1982). At about the same time, the placement staff at NTID/RIT was developing similar activities (Martin, 1982).

1975: *PL 94–142, the Education for All Handicapped Children Act*, required local education agencies to provide an appropriate education for all children in "the least restrictive environment." This Act brought more public attention to education for handicapped children. The effect of "least restrictive environment" interpretations has, in general, been bad for hearing-impaired students and their schools (Davila & Brill, 1976).

The National Center for Law and the Deaf (NCLD) began as an information and advisory service. It is located at Gallaudet College. NCLD's advent was especially timely because of extensive litigation arising from the Rehabilitation Act and PL 94–142. It also has helped awaken hearing-impaired people to their civil rights. More closely related to the focus of this study,

NCLD has encouraged a number of hearing-impaired persons to enter the profession of law (Dubow, 1983).

Regional Employment Seminar Programs were initiated at NTID to help firms learn to use hearing-impaired workers effectively. Fourteen of these seminars have been held with various firms since 1975 (Martin, 1982).

1976: *The Legal Defense Fund of the NAD* began to support litigation in key cases involving hearing-impaired persons. Hearing-impaired people have rarely used this civil rights tool (Dubow, 1983).

1978: *The Special School of the Future Project* involved the Kellogg Foundation, the Public Services Division of Gallaudet College, and five residential schools for the deaf. The project's aim was to promote the concept of the residential school for the deaf as a resource center for parent education, home-school relationships, curriculum development, continuing education for adults, and wider professional awareness (Special School of the Future, n.d.).

The National Center on Employment of the Deaf at NTID/RIT provides a focus for the extensive attention given there to technical training, career awareness, and placement. The center places much emphasis on employer information and development (Martin, 1982).

1980: *Southwest Collegiate Institute for the Deaf (SWCID)* was founded as a freestanding unit for higher education of hearing-impaired students. Although affiliated with Howard Junior College in Texas, the SWCID has its own campus (Crammatte, 1980).

Chapter One
THE PROFESSIONAL ENVIRONMENT

Research on the labor force related to professional employment is not confined merely to the job itself. Employees' socioeconomic status is of considerable relevance both to their backgrounds and work preparation and to their occupations, economic security, and participation in community and professional affairs.

In conducting the survey upon which this book is based, it was important to ask several relevant questions: Are these respondents truly professionals? Have their family backgrounds, education, and careers to date been those of typical professional workers? Are their occupations, salaries, and professional and community affiliations those expected of professional workers?

FAMILY STATUS

How can it be said that family socioeconomic status determines the direction a person may take occupationally? Parental expectations and the subtle influence of home environment probably influence occupational choice considerably. These factors are a part of what Jencks described as a "hypothetical variable" and are not really measurable directly. Measurable components of family socioeconomic status levels include parents' education, family size, neighborhood, schools, and economic status. All of these aspects relate closely to the occupational status of the father (and, in the past decade, of the mother). Hence, researchers use occupational status of the parent to represent the "hypothetical variable" (i.e., the socioeconomic status of the family).

Respondents were asked to name the usual, or more important, occupations of their parents when the respondents were "about age 16." The respondents also provided descriptions of the tasks their parents performed to aid in defining the occupations. Table 1 shows these occupations according to the classification used for the 1970 census (Bureau of the Census, 1971b). For comparison, Table 1 also includes similar occupational distributions from a national sample of

Table 1
Distribution of Occupational Categories Among
Parents of Hearing and Hearing-Impaired Children
(In %)

Occupation	Working Parents of Respondents Father	Working Parents of Respondents Mother	Parents of Hearing-Impaired Children[a] Father	Parents of Hearing-Impaired Children[a] Mother	Heads of Families United States Population[a] Male	Heads of Families United States Population[a] Female
Professional, Technical, and Kindred	20	22	16	15	14	15
Farmers and Farm Managers	7	1	3	—	3	1
Managers and Administrators	21	8	9	3	14	5
Clerical and Kindred	3	32	4	37	6	35
Sales	6	6	5	3	6	6
Crafts and Kindred	27	4	22	10	21	2
Operatives (including transportation)	9	14	19	9	18	13
Service	4	12	18	23	8	21
Farm Laborers	—	—	2	1	2	1
Laborers (except farm)	2	1	3	—	8	1
Total[b]	99	100	101	101	100	100

[a] The data in columns 2 and 3 are from *Two Studies of the Families of Hearing-Impaired Children* by B.W. Rawlings and C. J. Jensema, 1977. Washington, DC: Gallaudet College. Copyright 1977 by Gallaudet College. Adapted by permission.
[b] Discrepancies in totals are due to rounding.

"almost 800 families with one or more hearing impaired children enrolled in special educational programs" (Rawlings & Jensema, 1977) and the general U.S. population.

Table 1 shows that the parents of the hearing-impaired professionals surveyed were employed more often in professional, technical, and managerial work (males, 48%; females, 38%) than were the parents in the Rawlings and Jensema sample (males, 28%; females, 18%) or the general population (males, 31%; females, 21%). Also, the respondents' parents were less frequently reported as operatives, service workers, or laborers, (15% of the fathers, 27% of the mothers). Of respondents' mothers, 950, or 54.7%, were housewives. For the purposes of this survey, housewife was not considered an occupation, and so it was excluded from Table 1.

The Census Bureau's occupational classifications have been used since their inception for descriptive purposes, but they are too broad and heterogeneous for accurate scaling to measure socioeconomic status. O. D. Duncan (1961a, 1961b) devised a scale that relates socioeconomic status to occupational rank. This scale has been used to analyze deaf persons' employment progress (Duprez, 1971; Schroedel, 1976). (This scale is explained more fully in chap. 6). Other components of Jenck's "hypothetical variable" (neighborhood, residence, family size) relate closely to occupations and income. Scale scores range from a low of 1 to a high of 96, as shown in Table 2. [Note that all columns in Table 2 total 100%. In this table and subsequent tables, if columns do total 100%, then the totals do not appear in the table.]

Most scores above 60 on the Duncan scale result from professional, technical, and managerial occupations. In this range are 42.0% of the fathers of respondents as compared to 16.8% of the fathers of the National Census of the Deaf Population (NCDP; Schein & Delk, 1974) sample. The 40–59 range might be called nonprofessional white-collar workers, although some crafts workers are included. In this range, the proportions are closer: 20.4% of the survey group and 14.5% of the NCDP sample.

Scores below 40 indicate blue-collar workers. The respondents' fathers comprised 37.6% of this group, while the NCDP sample fathers made up 68.7% of that total.

From Tables 1 and 2 it can be said that the respondents came, as a rule, from families of higher than average socioeconomic status.

Jenck's "hypothetical variable" seems well established for this group of hearing-impaired professionals. Nevertheless, 957 (58%) of the respondents' working fathers scored below 60 on the Duncan scale. In contrast, 1701 (98%) of the respondents themselves scored at or above the 60 level. This indicates that a substantial number of the respondents have experienced the "American Dream" of upward social mobility. This aspect will be examined more closely in chapter 6.

ACADEMIC PREPARATION

Academic preparation is recognized as a predominant influence on career achievement. Jencks, Bartlett, et al. (1975) said that education accounts for about half of the explained variation in occupational status in the general population. Schroedel (1976/1977, 1982a, 1982b) found that this predominance also applies to deaf workers. He determined

Table 2
Socioeconomic Status of Fathers of Respondents and Fathers in National Census of the Deaf (NCDP) Sample
(In %)

Duncan Scale Scores	Fathers of Respondents $N=1650$	Fathers of NCDP Sample[a] $N=977$
90–96	4.4	0.6
80–89	8.1	2.2
70–79	7.9	3.0
60–69	21.6	11.0
50–59	13.2	7.6
40–49	7.2	6.9
30–39	7.1	6.9
20–29	7.7	9.3
10–19	20.7	44.0
1–9	2.1	8.5

Note. These classifications were used from 1940 to 1970. Extensive changes in classification, rank, and job titles were made for the 1980 census. In this study, the 1970 codes were used for the original coding and conversion to the Duncan scale. For descriptive data and current comparisons 1980 codes were used.

[a]The data in column 3 are from "Variables Related to the Attainment of Occupational Status Among Deaf Adults" by J. G. Schroedel, 1977, *DAI, 38*, p. 1048. Copyright 1977 by DAI. Adapted by permission.

that education had the highest correlation ($r = .46$) with occupational status in a sample from the National Census of the Deaf Population and in a group of National Technical Institute for the Deaf graduates ($r = .58$).

The respondents to the present survey were well prepared academically. Only 48 (2.8%) did not have some college education; 1605 (92.5%) had graduated from college, and 1065 (61.4%) had graduate degrees. How many more are still pursuing higher degrees is not known, for only degrees received were coded.

These figures are impressive, especially when compared with the 51.8% of the U.S. population of professional, technical, and managerial workers age 16 and over with comparable education (see Table 3). The lowest age included in the age range for the U.S. population data makes the figures not precisely comparable. The hearing-impaired respondents below age 25 number only 35, or 2% of the group, whereas workers below age 25 in the general population comprise 23% of the labor force. (This last statistic was not available for professional/managerial workers, just for the general population.) Revision of the U.S. professional/managerial population lowest age limit to 25 years would undoubtedly increase the proportion of those with 4 years or

Table 3
Highest Educational Level Completed by Respondents and Hearing Peers Age 16 and Over

Highest Educational Level Completed	Respondents Number	Respondents Percent	Employed Professional Workers in the U.S.[a] Percent
Less than twelfth grade	8	0.5	4.9
High school	40	2.3	22.4
Some college	81	4.7	20.9
BA/BS Degree	540	31.1	51.8[b]
MA/MS Degree	937	54.0	
Three-year Degree (J.D., M.Div., etc.)	36	2.1	
Doctorate	92	5.3	
Total	1734	100.0	100.0

[a] The data in column 3 are from *Educational Attainment of Workers, March 1982* by Bureau of Labor Statistics, 1983, Washington, DC: Department of Labor. Copyright 1983 by Department of Labor. Adapted by permission.
[b] These degrees were earned in 4 or more years.

more of college. However, an increase to 92.5%, as was found among the hearing-impaired professionals, is quite unlikely.

OCCUPATIONS AND ECONOMIC POSITION

The respondents to the present survey can be classified into 87 job titles. Table 4 shows the major occupational groupings and the number of respondents in each grouping. (See Appendix D for a detailed listing by job classification.)

Table 4
Current Occupations of Respondents

Type of Occupation	Respondents Number	Percent
Executive, administrative, and managerial occupations[a]	188	10.8
Management-related occupations[b]	177	10.2
Architects	7	0.4
Engineers, Surveyors, and Mapping Scientists	29	1.7
Mathematical and Computer Scientists	73	4.2
Natural Scientists	27	1.6
Health diagnosing occupations	11	0.6
Health assessment and treatment occupations	4	0.2
Teaching, postsecondary	97	5.6
Teaching, except postsecondary	677	38.9
Counselors, educational and vocational	131	7.6
Librarians, Archivists, and Curators	36	2.1
Social Scientists	24	1.4
Social and Recreational Workers	35	2.0
Religious Workers	31	1.8
Lawyers and Judges	8	0.5
Writers, Artists, Entertainers, and Athletes	70	4.0
Health Technologists and Technicians	28	1.6
Engineering and related Technologists and Technicians	21	1.2
Science Technicians	1	0.1
Other Technicians	60	3.5
Total	1735	100.0

[a]This category includes 145 respondents in education or other service to deaf people.
[b]This category includes 23 respondents in education or other service to deaf people.

The great majority of the respondents held positions in educational institutions (1091, or 63%). The bulk of the remaining respondents worked in government (17.8%) and private business (14.4%). The remaining categories include self-employment (2.3%), religious organizations (2.0%), and hospitals (0.5%). Three respondents did not state their employer classification. Table 5 indicates that these hearing-impaired professionals earn salaries comparable to, but generally lower than, those earned by other professional workers. The median salary of respondents was $21,957. This is a little bit less than the $23,663 median *money income* (i.e., income from all sources—salaries, self-employment, social security or other retirement benefits, SSI, interest, dividends, and regular contributions from persons not living in the household) reported for managerial, professional specialty, and technical workers by the Census Bureau (Welniak & Henson, 1984). Since money income includes sources other than salaries, the hearing-impaired professional appears to be well paid.

There is another form of income available to working people, and that is *psychic income* (i.e., the pleasure they find in their daily occupations). This can be a large reward for the professional worker; when jobs are challenging, they can be quite satisfying. To attempt to measure this very subjective element, respondents were asked to

Table 5
Comparison of Salary Income of Respondents and
Money Income of Hearing Peers

Salary	Respondents Number	Respondents Percent	General Population Age 15 and Over[a] Percent
Under $10,000	46	2.7	6.8
10,000–19,999	675	39.5	32.5
20,000–29,999	687	40.2	29.3
30,000–39,999	218	12.7	15.2
40,000–49,999	57	3.3	6.9
50,000 and over	28	1.6	9.3
Total	1711	100.0	100.0

[a]The data in column 3 are from *Money Income of Households, Families, and Persons in the United States: 1982* by E.J. Welniak and M.F. Henson, 1984, Washington, DC: Bureau of the Census. Copyright 1984 by Bureau of the Census. Adapted by permission.

Table 6
Job Satisfaction as Perceived by Respondents
(In %)

	Job Satisfaction					
Degree of Liking	Chances for Promotion n=1665	Kind of work n=1714	Supervisors n=1703	Colleagues n=1696	Subordinates n=1655	Salary n=1702
Like very much	39.0	79.9	61.9	73.7	51.1	42.2
Like a little	16.2	14.1	23.1	19.0	11.8	34.4
Dislike a little	5.1	4.3	6.6	2.4	1.6	13.5
Dislike very much	5.0	1.3	3.4	0.5	0.8	8.6
Does not apply	34.7	0.4	5.0	4.4	34.7	1.3
Index of job satisfaction	0.79	1.67	1.33	1.63	1.11	0.88

rate six factors in the work situation. Their responses are shown in Table 6.

Table 6 shows only two categories where less than half of the respondents did not report "like very much"—salary and chances for promotion. Not many human beings are overjoyed about their salaries, so this answer is not so unexpected. The "chances for promotion" answer, however, may have been affected by the large number (a bit over one third) of respondents who said that this query was not applicable to their jobs. These replies came, for the most part, from classroom teachers. (See Appendix F for another type of data analysis.)

There is another measure of job satisfaction for hearing-impaired persons—discrimination. Considerable dimming of job satisfaction can occur if there is, or has been, unfair rejection in the workplace, no matter how much the worker may like the work itself. Yet, the 1960 study found that only 20% of the respondents had experienced discrimination, and that occurred chiefly at the hiring stage.

In the present study, respondents were asked, "How often have you experienced unfair rejection by employers in each of the job activities listed below?" Their answers were limited to a five-level scale ranging from "never" to "very often." The results are shown in Table 7.

More than 40% of the respondents reported never having experienced unfair rejection except in the case of communication, which 32%

Table 7
Extent of Rejection Perceived by Respondents
(In %)

Perceived Degree of Rejection	Hiring $n=1629$	Promotion $n=1571$	Training $n=1600$	Evaluation $n=1640$	Communication $n=1648$	Salary $n=1614$
Never	41.9	43.7	53.9	45.4	32.0	43.5
Almost never	20.0	20.3	20.3	25.0	22.3	22.0
Sometimes	24.7	23.0	17.2	20.4	30.9	24.2
Often	8.3	8.7	6.4	6.5	9.2	7.2
Very often	5.1	4.3	2.2	2.7	5.6	3.1
Index of discrimination	1.15	1.09	0.83	0.96	1.34	1.04

did report. A little over 10% did say that they had experienced rejection often or very often. Again, the frequency of rejection was greatest for communication. Nevertheless, more than half of the respondents almost never or never at all perceived unfair rejection in relation to their jobs.

Another way of analyzing the figures is by using indexes. Calculation of indexes of rejection is shown in Appendix F. The resultant indexes vary from 0 (never) to 4 (very often). The indexes shown in Table 7 indicate that almost no unfair rejection was perceived by the respondents.

PROFESSIONAL AFFILIATION

The true professional, aware of the obligation to keep abreast of developments in one's field, is a member of one or more professional associations. Those respondents working in the deaf sector (see definitions, p. 189) have several professional groups available to them, such as the Convention of American Instructors of the Deaf, the Conference of Educational Administrators Serving the Deaf, the A. G. Bell Association, the American Deafness and Rehabilitation Association, and the Registry of Interpreters for the Deaf.

Respondents working in the hearing sector, however, do not easily reap the benefits of professional affiliation (ideas, discussions with peers, grapevine news of new openings or new discoveries in the field). All of these require hearing, as distinguished from speech skills; these social interchanges and informal technical discussions often occur in group situations where even the best speechreader may be at a loss.

Special interest groups or sections in professional organizations might lower this barrier to a degree. However, a special interest group implies a substantial number of active members and an interest which relates deafness to the professional discipline in some way. If these conditions are not present, it becomes just a social adjunct to the parent organization.

The respondents' membership and participation in professional societies is reported in Table 8. The percentage of respondents who belonged to one or more professional societies was 65.2. Only 83 (4.8%) of the total group of 1,735 belonged to five or more professional associations. A scant few reported belonging to more than five; however, the questionnaire did not ask that question.

More than half of the one-organization group were active members: 61.2% of the members participated in one or more of the group's activities (e.g., attendance at meetings, committee work, or holding office).

COMMUNITY PARTICIPATION

One way to measure a person's standing in the community is to find out how other members of the community regard that person. That the 1982 respondents were held in high esteem was initially shown by the

Table 8
Professional Affiliations and Participation
(In %)

Participation	One $n=1132$	Two $n=740$	Three $n=439$	Four $n=218$	Five $n=83$
Inactive (paid dues)	38.8	39.6	35.1	31.2	26.5
One activity	36.0	35.6	39.1	44.9	36.1
Two activities	15.7	18.6	16.2	16.1	24.1
Three activities	9.5	6.2	9.6	7.8	13.3

Table 9
Participation in Community Organizations
(In %)

Participation	One n=1304	Two n=1017	Three n=663	Four n=356	Five n=132
	\multicolumn{5}{c}{Number of Organizations Joined}
Inactive (paid dues)	26.3	21.2	18.9	18.9	22.7
One activity	28.6	31.3	30.7	30.5	25.8
Two activities	20.9	23.8	24.0	22.8	25.0
Three activities	24.2	23.7	26.4	27.8	26.5

fact that they were named in lists and by knowledgeable people as professional workers. Another measure of community acceptance is the extent to which the respondents participated in community affairs. In the context of this study, community affairs included state and national organizations of hearing-impaired people as well as local groups.

Table 9 shows the number of organizations to which the respondents belonged. It also shows the extent of their activeness in the organizations. A total of 1,304 (75.2%) respondents were members of at least one community organization; of these, 26.3% were inactive dues-paying members; 28.6% were engaged in one activity, in most cases attending meetings; 20.9% participated in two activities, mainly meetings and committee service; and 24.2% were involved in three activities, such as meetings, committees, offices.

The number of respondents who were members of more than one community organization declined as the number of organizations to which they belonged increased. One hundred thirty-two of the respondents (7.6%) belonged to five organizations. Of these, 35 had been engaged in three activities.

Summary

Looking at the 1982 respondents as a whole, they do meet the qualifications for being classified as true professionals. These qualifications can be listed as follows:
1. A comparatively high percentage have or had parents in professional or managerial occupations.

2. They are, in the main, highly educated.
3. They are employed in managerial, professional, or technical occupations.
4. They earn a median salary of $21,957 (this figure is somewhat less than the median salary for professional peers who hear).
5. They appear to be reasonably well satisfied with their jobs, having experienced very little unfair rejection.
6. Their professional and community service affiliations are fairly high; a majority of persons so affiliated have participated actively in various organizations.

Chapter Two
COMMUNICATION

It is a well-known fact that the ability to communicate is an important component in the lives of all people. In situations that do not require communication, a hearing impairment can go unnoticed. This invisibleness can lead people not familiar with deafness to underestimate its ramifications.

Hearing impairment affects family relations, education, employment, and social relations; in other words, all areas of a hearing-impaired person's life. The problems of communication are so pervasive that they affect practically all of the analyses attempted in this study. Yet communication has aspects that can be examined by themselves; these aspects will be explored in this chapter. The relation of communication difficulties to the job, work satisfaction, discrimination, and professional affiliation will be approached in later chapters.

Hearing-impaired people vary in their use of different communication modes. The variations ranged, in this survey, from the 71 respondents (4.1%) who reported that they do not use sign language, through the great majority who use signs and speech as appropriate, to those 191 (11.0%) who do not use speech at all.

There are numerous professional positions that do not require that communication be conducted by speech alone. One of the largest groups of these professionals is teachers at schools for deaf children. Other positions for which sign language fluency is an asset include rehabilitation counselors (Degrell & Ouelette, 1981); psychological service workers (Spragins, Karchmer, & Schildroth, 1981); social workers; and administrative personnel such as program directors or coordinators, principals, and heads of schools for deaf children.

Many of the respondents in this survey reported that they work in positions that do not require speech all the time: 1,091 work in educational institutions (presumably, in most cases, for hearing-impaired persons); 130 work in rehabilitation or school counseling offices. A few are actors who use their skill at signs, mime, and body language to great effect on the stage and screen. Some work in government agencies concerned with deafness.

A substantial percentage of the respondents (about 23%) work in private industry, government agencies, or their own businesses where oral communication is absolutely necessary. Their deafness is not an asset as far as work is concerned.

The emphasis in this chapter is on speech and speechreading because that is where the majority of communication problems occur. The main concern in the survey was how the respondents communicated with hearing co-workers and how effective this communication was. To find out this information, the respondents were asked to check their most frequently used mode of communication with hearing co-workers: writing, talking, sign language without speech, sign language with speech, fingerspelling only, and other means. Table 10 shows the frequency with which these modes were used.

Sign language (with and without speech) was the most frequently used means of communication with hearing co-workers; 45.9% use that mode for expression and 48.8% use it for reception. If other, similar categories in Table 10 (*fingerspelling, at a school for the deaf*, and *when using an interpreter*) are added to the sign language classifications, the percentages increase to 46.4 and 50.2 respectively. These proportions probably result from the many respondents who work in educational institutions. Talking was the next most frequently used category; 41.1% of the respondents use speech and 36.7% use speechreading. Over 100 respondents gave multiple responses to this question—*talking and sign language* was the most common; however, multiple responses were excluded from the table.

Table 10
Means of Communication
Used Most Frequently with Hearing Co-workers

	Respondents			
	Expressive		Receptive	
Means of Communication	Number	Percent	Number	Percent
Writing	200	12.5	210	13.1
Talking[a]	661	41.1	591	36.7
Sign language without speech	143	8.9	58	3.6
Sign language with speech	594	37.0	726	45.2
Fingerspelling only	3	0.2	8	0.5
Uses an interpreter	5	0.3	4	0.2
Works in school for the deaf[b]	—	—	12	0.7
Total	1606	100.0	1609	100.0

[a]*Talking* means speechreading for reception.
[b]This category was included because respondents were able to use whatever means of communication was suitable at a given time.

How a person communicates in a hearing environment depends largely upon his or her speech skills. It is important to remember that the survey respondents' assessment of their own speech skills was based on their self-perceptions. In the previous study (Crammatte, 1968), co-workers rated respondents' speech more highly than did the respondents themselves, especially as regards reception. Table 11 shows how the respondents rated their speech skills. The table also shows the proportion of daily communication that respondents perceive as being with co-workers who do not use sign language.

Interpreting the results in Table 11 requires a careful look at the second level of speech skill (see Appendix C). Several ambiguous words were used in the survey: *almost, often, short*, and *carefully*. The respondents no doubt read different meanings into these words. The intent at the second skill level was to show a level of speech and speechreading that is less than fluent (i.e., conversation that stumbles and may be strained, but does communicate in an oral mode.)

Elsewhere in this report (chapter 6) the speech skills are reclassified as *good, fair*, and *poor*. It may be helpful to the reader to keep that interpretation in mind. It will also be wise to remember that the respondents' evaluations were completely subjective.

If the two highest classifications of speech skills are taken to represent usable oral communication, it seems that as the need for oral communication increases (i.e., more need for communication with nonsigners) so does the proportion of respondents having these higher speech skills, an obvious conclusion.

Except for this conclusion, the respondents showed very little variation in speech skills for the different degrees of oral communication. As a group, they also rated their perception of their receptive skills lower than their expressive skills at every level. In other words, most respondents have more confidence in their speech than in their speechreading.

Looking at the data from a different point of view, about five eighths of this group communicate at work less than half the time with people who do not use sign language (1017, or 61.8%, expressively and 1082, or 62.5%, receptively).

Different proportions of the respondents communicate socially with people who do not use sign language. The percentage of re-

Table 11
Use of Expressive and Receptive Speech Skills at Work
With People Who Do Not Sign
(In %)

Speech Skills	0–24%	25–49%	50–74%	75–100%	Total
Expressive	$n=762$	$n=255$	$n=186$	$n=442$	$N=1645$
Co-workers understand					
Almost all said	46.8	45.9	58.5	64.7	52.7
Almost all but must repeat	27.0	38.8	31.2	27.6	29.5
Word or two now and then	19.4	10.2	6.5	5.9	12.9
Does not use speech[a]	6.8	5.1	3.8	1.8	4.9
Receptive	$n=791$	$n=261$	$n=189$	$n=441$	$N=1682$
Respondent understands					
Almost all said	36.5	34.5	43.5	55.6	42.0
Short conversation, with care	28.6	40.6	39.1	35.6	33.5
Short sentence	18.2	13.4	10.6	5.4	13.2
Does not use speechreading[a]	16.7	11.5	6.8	3.4	11.3

[a]This category includes: "I do not use speech," 59; "work at school for the deaf," 15; and "use an interpreter," 6.

spondents who communicate less than half of the time with nonsigners was 62.9%, whereas 37.1% reported communicating more than half the time with people who do not sign.

These data pose another question, one not covered by this study—Did having higher speech skills induce some respondents to enter positions in oral environments (50–100% level), or did they retain and improve their speech skills because they used them daily at work?

The extent of hearing impairment is a significant factor in assessing speech skills. Obviously, the less than severely impaired person has enough residual hearing either to function in certain situations or to be helped by a hearing aid. Often sufficient hearing to recognize tones and variations in speech will be of help in speechreading. The profoundly impaired person often has no viable residual hearing acuity.

Table 12 shows the relationship between speech skills and extent of hearing impairment. The highest skill, "almost all said," is predominant among respondents whose impairment is less than severe. (Classification of extent of impairment is explained in Appendix B.) Of the less than severely impaired, 79.9% could speak clearly enough for

Table 12
A Comparison of Expressive and Receptive Speech Skills
By Extent of Impairment
(In %)

Speech Skills	Less Than Severe	Severe	Profound	Total
Expressive	$n=340$	$n=299$	$n=1015$	$N=1654$
Co-workers understand				
Almost all said	79.9	45.2	45.9	52.8
Almost all, but must repeat	17.1	36.5	31.6	29.5
Word or two now and then	1.5	14.0	16.4	12.9
Does not use speech	1.5	4.3	6.1	4.8
Receptive	$n=339$	$n=306$	$n=1045$	$N=1690$
Respondent understands				
Almost all said	68.1	40.2	33.9	41.9
Short conversation, with care	25.4	36.9	35.1	33.5
Short sentence	4.7	12.4	16.4	13.3
Does not use speechreading	1.8	10.5	14.6	11.3

co-workers to understand almost all they said without difficulty; 68.1% of them could receive speech with the same facility. On the other hand, only about 32 to 36% of the severely and profoundly impaired could carry on an extended conversation. This difference probably arises from the fact that some of the less than severely impaired can hear well enough to converse, while others gain clues for speechreading from what they do hear. However, it must be remembered that partial hearing can cause distortions that may make understanding difficult.

Age of occurrence of hearing impairment also affects speech skills. The person who became hearing impaired after acquiring speech in the usual auditory manner is likely to use speech expressively more readily and with greater confidence than someone who has never heard speech and so has had to learn it by a most laborious process. Such is not always the case for speech reception. Perhaps that is because some persons who once could hear have not gone through the long, arduous process of learning to speechread. The relationships between age of occurrence and speech skills are considered in Table 13.

Table 13
Expressive and Receptive Speech Skills
By Age When Impairment Occurred
(In %)

| Speech Skills | _____Age When Impairment Occurred_____ | | | | |
	0–2	3–5	6–11	12 and over	Total
Expressive	$n=1141$	$n=195$	$n=167$	$n=133$	$N=1636$
Co-workers understand					
Almost all said	42.7	69.3	72.5	90.2	52.8
Almost all but must repeat	34.8	17.9	23.9	9.8	29.6
Word or two now and then	16.3	8.7	3.6	—	12.8
Does not use speech	6.2	4.1	—	—	4.8
Receptive	$n=1172$	$n=200$	$n=167$	$n=132$	$N=1671$
Respondent understands					
Almost all said	40.9	48.5	43.7	40.2	42.0
Short conversation, with care	32.0	30.0	38.9	43.1	33.3
Short sentences	14.9	13.0	6.6	7.6	13.3
Does not use speechreading	12.2	8.5	10.8	9.1	11.4

As might be expected, less than half of the respondents who became hearing impaired before age 3 ranked their speech skills at the highest level. About three fourths saw themselves as having either of the two highest levels. Age 6 appears to be the dividing line where the proportion of the orally fluent rises. Of those impaired after age 12, 90% speak fluently, but only 40% have top receptive skills. Receptive skills are fairly similar for all ages of impairment.

Speech skills are not the only communication skills affected by age of occurrence. Linguists say that the first 3 years of life are crucial to the acquisition of language (Brown, 1973). Children whose hearing is impaired before age 3 face barriers to developing fluency in a verbal language, especially because they are denied the countless auditory stimuli necessary for language learning. Every word must be learned through vision and, in most cases, must have been deliberately taught. The importance of verbal skill to subsequent learning, especially to higher learning of professional theory and technique, is obvious.

Communication barriers can also interfere with family bonding. Deaf babies in hearing families often are neglected, or, maybe worse, overprotected. Yet some persons whose hearing became profoundly impaired before age 3 have overcome these substantial barriers and have achieved professional status.

Of the respondents that reported age of occurrence, 70.2% became hearing impaired before age 3 (see Table 14). This datum supports the following finding of the 1960 study of deaf professionals: "In

Table 14
Age of Occurrence and Extent of Hearing Impairment
(In %)

Age of Occurrence	Less Than Severe n=337	Severe n=311	Profound n=1063	Total N=1711
Less than 1 year	49.6	60.2	55.8	55.4
1–2 years	16.6	19.3	12.9	14.8
3–5 years	13.6	10.9	11.7	11.9
6–11 years	9.2	5.1	11.8	10.1
12–18 years	3.9	1.9	4.5	3.9
19 years and over	7.1	2.6	3.3	3.9

short this finding (that 30 percent of the respondents had been born deaf) denies a too prevalent negative attitude that a person born deaf is so deeply handicapped that significant educational and professional accomplishment is not possible" (Crammatte, 1968).

Fluency in sign language is not a major concern of this study. Except for professionals working with deaf persons (e.g., as teachers, social workers, counselors, etc.), fluency in manual communication is not a critical factor. An exception is acting, where mime and body language are vital for hearing-impaired actors and actresses.

A great deal of attention has been given in this chapter to skills in speech and speechreading. These skills have been emphasized because they are the major source of problems in the workplace. Communication can be severely hindered when one party uses a language based on sound and the other uses a language that is visual. When a visible communication mode is appropriate (e.g., when working with other hearing-impaired persons), then sign language becomes a solution, not a problem.

It is of interest to know from whom the respondents learned to sign. This information reveals indirectly whether sign language can be called a *native language*; that is, the mode of communication that was learned as a child from parents, siblings, friends, or classmates. Respondents were asked, "From whom did you first learn to sign?" Their choices were school friends, college friends, family, friends outside of school, and school staff or teachers. Using these categories, a sizable majority of the respondents (72.1%) appear to be native signers. A mere 6% reported learning from school personnel—rare is the school for the deaf that teaches deaf people's language.

Summary

A majority of the survey respondents are in occupations serving deaf people. For them, communication difficulties at work are rare. Examination of communication modes used and the speech skills involved indicates that those who need oral communication at work are reasonably proficient in its use. A majority of the respondents socialize mainly with people who use sign language, which is a first language for most respondents.

Speech skills are affected by the severity of the impairment and the age when it occurred. The less than severely impaired appear better able to communicate orally. Of those impaired before speech was well established (about age 6), a large proportion did learn to speak and read lips. However, the proportion able to communicate by speech rises rapidly among those deafened after age 6. For speechreading, the proportions are about the same for each age group.

More will be considered in later chapters about means of communication and their relation to situations at work and in professional and community associations.

Chapter Three
EDUCATION

The field of education of hearing-impaired persons is a complex and fascinating one. It includes a variety of educational settings and a surprising breadth and depth of difficulties and problems.

The importance of education to a professional career is a well-established fact. The very definition of a profession includes "the study of a theoretical structure of a department of learning" (Carr-Saunders, 1955). College education is also widely recognized as a predictor of professional occupation and socioeconomic status (Jencks, Bartlett, et al., 1975). In addition, education, and therefore professional competence, aids in overcoming employment barriers arising from a hearing impairment (e.g., low expectations and reluctance to employ).

Education of hearing-impaired children involves a variety of school settings. Table 15 shows the types of schools from which respondents received their high school diplomas. The preponderance of graduates from residential schools (52.2%) is to be expected. Data on high school graduates from special educational facilities for hearing-impaired students show more than half from residential schools in 1982 and prior years (Craig & Craig, 1983). The proportions demonstrated in Table 15 are similar to those from previous years.

The more remarkable finding in Table 15 is the small proportion of respondents who received their high school diplomas from general schools with programs for deaf students (5.8%). Data on special education facilities show that almost 39% of all high school graduates come from *day classes*, the classification comparable to *general, with special programs* in Table 15 (Craig & Craig, 1983). The discrepancy between 5.8% and 39% probably can be explained by the 41.7% of respondents graduated from general high schools and boarding schools. Special day classes generally encourage students to go on to general high schools upon completion of their elementary schooling.

The 1982 study of deaf professionals made no attempt to find the type of elementary school attended by the respondents. The only question about precollege education asked from what type of educational institution they had received their high school diplomas.

Day classes, the other school setting with numerous graduates, provided only 5.8% of these professional workers. This situation can probably be explained by the fact that this type of educational institution has tended to move students into regular high schools whenever possible. The data in Table 15 for general high schools with no special program support this idea.

As might be expected, persons with severe and profound hearing impairments tended to gravitate toward schools with special programs for such children. Of the 1,377 respondents with severe and profound

Table 15
Type of High School from Which Respondents Graduated

Type of High School	Respondents Number	Percent
Residential school for hearing-impaired students	872	50.7
Day school for hearing-impaired students	25	1.5
General, with program for hearing-impaired students	99	5.8
General	627	36.4
Boarding school	81	4.7
Other[a]	6	0.3
No high school diploma	10	0.6
Total	1720	100.0

[a]This category includes correspondence school, 3; high school equivalency examination, 2; tutor, 1.

impairments, 56.0% attended residential programs; 31.2% graduated from high schools with no special program.

Conversely, most of the 341 respondents with less than severe impairment had attended general educational institutions—58.4% graduated from general public high schools with no special programs, whereas only 28.4% graduated from residential schools for the deaf.

It is quite probable that the proportion of hearing-impaired graduates of general high schools with special programs will increase in future years. This will happen as a result of Public Law 94-142, the legislative spur to *mainstreaming* (i.e., enrolling handicapped children in public school programs). The quality of education in that setting versus that of the residential school is a matter of controversy, one that will not be resolved for a number of years, if ever.

Age of occurrence of hearing impairment also seems to have been related to choice of school. Of the 861 respondents who reported both age of impairment and graduation from a residential school, 78.0% lost their hearing before age 3; only 11.4% lost their hearing after age 6. Of the 698 who attended high schools without a special program, 59.6% became hearing impaired before age 3 and 27.5% after age 6. Almost 34% of those who became hearing impaired before age 3 received diplomas from high schools with no special program for hearing-impaired students.

The proportion of students graduating from general public high schools rises with each age group. The highest number of graduates from public schools is found in the age group of 12 and older. In this group, 110, or 83.3%, graduated from public schools with no special programs. No respondents deafened after age 6 received high school diplomas from day schools. This finding is not surprising in view of the practice of many day schools of urging eighth-grade graduates to continue in general high schools.

The relationship of type of high school to highest educational attainment provides some interesting information. At the baccalaureate and master's levels, more respondents had received their high school diplomas from residential schools for the deaf—over 50%—than from general programs—less than 40%. At the doctoral level, 55.2% had graduated from general high schools with no special program for deaf students as compared to 28.1% from residential schools for the deaf. The heavy concentration of respondents in the MA/MS group (933, or

54%) is probably due in part to the certification requirements for the many teachers in the study. Of course, the fact that someone graduated from a certain type of high school does not necessarily mean that he or she attended that sort of school for his or her entire education.

It should be noted that the level of education attained is understated in these data. A number of respondents were engaged in graduate study beyond the degree they reported. These added attainments were ignored because degree actually earned was a more objective figure than midcourse attainment. A few of those included at the MA/MS level who are personally known to the researcher have completed their doctorates since the time they completed the survey.

Level of education attained plays an important role in the professional employment of hearing-impaired people. Schroedel (1976/1977), in his study of the national census of the deaf population (NCDP), found level of education to be the strongest predictor of occupational status ($r = .46, p < .001$). This relationship may not be so readily measured with the present data as with the NCDP sample. The NCDP sample covered all areas of employment, whereas those in the present group were by definition all professionally employed.

In most cases, a college degree is a necessary credential for professional appointment, especially for a person with a disability (see Table 3 and pp. 16–18). The data seem to indicate that, for people with a hearing impairment, a graduate degree is very helpful in achieving

Table 16
Highest Educational Level Attained
By Age of Occurrence of Hearing Impairment
(In %)

Highest Educational Level Attained	Less Than 3 Years $n=1203$	3–5 Years $n=204$	6–11 Years $n=171$	12 Years and Older $n=134$	Total $N=1712$
No College Degree	8.4	7.4	5.8	2.2	7.5
Bachelor's Degree	35.2	26.0	22.8	14.2	31.2
Master's Degree	51.5	57.2	57.3	64.9	53.9
3-Year Degree[a]	1.2	2.5	5.3	4.5	2.0
Doctorate	3.7	6.9	8.8	14.2	5.4

[a]This category includes J.D. and D.Div. degrees.

professional or managerial status. As can be seen from Table 16, 7.5% of the respondents did not reach the BA/BS level; however, 1,049 (over 60%) had at least a master's degree.

The data also show that persons deafened after age 12 earned more advanced degrees than those impaired before age 3. These figures are, however, distorted by the fact that there are so many respondents whose impairment occurred before age 3 (1203, or about 70%). Looking at the doctorates from another perspective, of the 92 earned, 44 (47.8%) went to persons impaired before age 3.

There is a much less significant relationship between attainment of graduate degrees and level of hearing impairment. Extent of impairment apparently did not affect the highest college degree earned. The proportion of respondents at the various levels of attainment is quite similar for each level of impairment.

Another aspect of communication related to educational attainment is a hearing-impaired person's degree of oral skills. It would seem that oral skills (both expressive and receptive) are a help to those who seek educational attainment. This is especially true at the graduate level because few colleges provide the necessary special services to alleviate communication difficulties. This, of course, is not the case at specialized institutions such as Gallaudet College.

Respondents rated their oral expressive and receptive skills higher as their level of academic attainment increased (see Table 17). The proportion of doctoral degree holders claiming top receptive skills is quite large (73.9%). Surprisingly, 15.6% of this same group of respondents do not use speech.

The previous study conducted in 1960 examined in some depth the problems that severely and profoundly deaf professional workers had experienced in pursuing advanced study (Crammatte, 1968). These problems included taking lecture notes, attending seminars, consulting with professors, asking questions in class, and meeting requirements in speech or foreign language classes. All of these difficulties still remain; however, they have been alleviated to some extent by support services that did not exist at all in 1960.

The present study asked only about the services provided for hearing-impaired students by some general colleges and universities. For this reason, the responses of the 406 professionals who had attended Gallaudet or the National Technical Institute for the Deaf

Table 17
Expressive and Receptive Speech Skills
By Highest Educational Level Attained
(In %)

Speech Skills	No College Degree	Bachelor's Degree	Master's Degree	3-year Degree	Doctorate	Total
Expressive	n=121	n=529	n=914	n=35	n=90	N=1689
Co-workers understand						
Almost all said	41.4	38.8	42.7	57.1	49.9	42.0
Almost all but must repeat	32.2	38.0	31.3	34.3	28.9	33.4
Word or two now and then	19.8	13.6	13.1	8.6	5.6	13.3
Respondent does not use speech	6.6	9.6	12.9	0	15.6	11.3
Receptive	n=123	n=512	n=895	n=35	n=88	N=1653
Respondent understands						
Almost all said	34.1	44.8	57.2	68.5	73.9	52.8
Short conversation	39.1	35.4	26.1	25.7	18.2	29.5
Short sentence	18.7	13.9	12.5	2.9	6.8	12.9
Respondent does not use speechreading	8.1	5.9	4.2	2.9	1.1	4.8

(NTID/RIT) as undergraduates were not counted. However, if they had taken graduate courses at other institutions, then their responses were included.

According to the respondents, the most frequently available support service was the help of notetakers (see Table 18). The 1960 study mentioned some ingenious means to the end of securing notes, such as providing carbon paper and typing out classmates' notes. In the mid-1960s, NTID/RIT developed notetaker paper that produced copies without the need for carbon paper.

Providing interpreters is a fairly new service at colleges and universities. This practice was mandated by amendments to the Rehabilitation Act of 1973. Lawsuits demanding this service occurred in the late 1970s.

Table 19 shows the respondents' major areas of concentration during their undergraduate years. Considering that 1,076 of them are

Table 18
Support Services Available to Respondents
At Regular Colleges and Universities

Support Service	Respondents Number	Percent
Notetakers	860	64.7
Interpreters	773	58.2
Favorable seating	475	35.7
Copies of notes provided	360	27.1
Professors who knew about deafness	327	29.6
Speech and hearing center	89	6.7
Tutors	80	6.0
Attendance at classes not required	74	5.6
Counselors	72	5.4

Note. The total number of responses for all support services exceeds the total number of respondents because many gave multiple answers. 406 respondents had attended only Gallaudet College or NTID, where communication is tailored to hearing-impaired students.

employed by educational institutions, it may seem peculiar that only 278 majored in education (either regular education, elementary education, special education, or physical education). This apparent anomaly is explained by the fact that for about 20 years, Gallaudet College (source of the bachelor's degree for 1,052 respondents) had no education major. Students took humanities or the behavioral sciences to prepare for graduate study in education.

Many hearing-impaired children spend more years obtaining their education than do normally hearing children. Some schools have as many as three preparatory years, and some keep children until they are as old as 21. Also, Gallaudet has its preparatory year and NTID/RIT its vestibule courses. Therefore, it is not too surprising that more than one third of the respondents received their baccalaureate degrees somewhat later in life than the general population of college students. Table 20 shows the respondents' distribution of ages at graduation.

Most of the respondents (1,052, or 60.6%) received their bachelor's degrees from Gallaudet College. This preponderance may have resulted from the fact that a listing of Gallaudet graduates in professional work provided the base for the survey mailing list. Also, Gallaudet is much older than any of the other collegiate programs for hearing-impaired persons. There are two other special baccalaureate

Table 19
Undergraduate Areas of Major Concentration
Reported by 10 or More Respondents

Major Concentration	Number of Respondents
Accounting	37
American Studies	13
Art/Fine Arts	40
Biological Sciences	60
Business Administration	93
Chemistry and Chemical Engineering Technology	51
Communication	10
Economics	19
Education	129
Elementary Education	29
English	148
History	76
Home Economics	61
Liberal Arts	54
Library Science	51
Mathematics	138
Philosophy	12
Physical Education	72
Physics	12
Physiology	16
Political Science	11
Psychology	114
Social Work	51
Sociology	82
Special Education	48
Total	1427

institutions—NTID, from which 53 respondents had graduated; and California State University, Northridge (CSUN), from which 9 respondents had graduated. The remaining respondents had BA/BS degrees from various other colleges and universities (a total of 489, or 28.2% of the whole group).

It is evident from Table 21 that in the 1960s and 1970s increasing numbers of hearing-impaired people took advantage of the new opportunities for higher education. The largest number of respondents (264)

Table 20
Respondents' Age Upon Receipt of Bachelor's Degree

Age	Respondents Number	Percent
Less than 20	14	0.9
20–24	1002	63.5
25–29	425	27.0
30–34	58	3.7
35–39	30	1.9
40–44	29	1.8
45–49	9	0.6
50 and over	9	0.6
Total	1576	100.0

Note. 159 respondents did not report year of graduation.

graduated with bachelor's degrees in 1974–1976. The number of graduates decreases radically after 1980, probably because potential professionals are in graduate school or are working up the ladder to professional status.

How well educated are these hearing-impaired people in professional or managerial positions as compared to their peers in the United States population? From Table 22, it is obvious that the hearing-impaired respondents are better educated than the general population of professional/managerial workers. Of course the U.S. population figures are pulled downward by that portion of the population age 16 to 22 (the youngest hearing-impaired respondent was 22). However, there cannot be many of this age group among professional workers (5.6% of

Table 21
Respondents by Year of Graduation from Undergraduate Programs

Year of Graduation	Respondents Number	Percent
1943 or earlier	40	2.5
1944–1953	156	9.9
1954–1963	237	15.0
1964–1973	620	39.2
1974–1983	529	33.4
Total	1582	100.0

Table 22
Highest Educational Level Attained by Respondents and
Hearing Peers Age 16 and Over
(In %)

Highest Educational Level	Respondents N=1710	Hearing Professional/ Managerial Workers N=28,432,000 [a]
Grade 12 or less	2.8	27.3
Some college	4.7	20.9
Bachelors degree or higher	92.5	51.8

[a]The data in column 3 are from *Educational Attainment of Workers, March 1982* by Bureau of Labor Statistics, 1983, Washington, DC: Department of Labor. Copyright 1983 by Department of Labor. Adapted by permission.

all working families, regardless of occupation, were in the 15–24 year age group [Welniak & Henson, 1984]).

Given that this group is well educated, are they reimbursed in proportion to their education? Tables 23 and 24 examine different aspects of this question.

The median salary earned by respondents was $21,957. Taking $20,000 as a point of separation, the breakdown of salaries over $20,000 based on level of education is as follows:

Grade 12 or less: 57.4%   MA/MS: 59.7%
Some College: 38.0%   3-year degree: 63.9%
BA/BS: 50.7%   Doctorate   95.6%

Table 23
Salary by Highest Educational Level Attained
(In %)

	Highest Educational Level						
Salary	Grade 12 or less n=47	Some College n=79	Bachelor's Degree n=531	Master's Degree n=925	3-Year Degree n=36	Doctorate n=92	Total N=1710
Less than $10,000	2.1	1.3	4.1	1.8	11.1	1.1	2.7
$10,000–$19,999	40.5	60.7	45.3	38.5	25.0	3.3	39.5
$20,000–$29,999	34.1	31.6	33.3	46.1	36.1	32.6	40.2
$30,000–$39,999	19.1	3.8	12.8	11.0	13.9	32.6	12.7
$40,000–$49,999	2.1	1.3	3.6	2.1	5.6	16.3	3.3
$50,000 and over	2.1	1.3	0.9	0.5	8.3	14.1	1.6

Table 24
Relation of Educational Attainment to Median Salaries of
Respondents and Median Money Income of
Persons 25 Years Old and Over

Median Salary or Income	Highest Educational Level			
	Grade 12 or less	Some College	4 Years College	5 Years College or more
Respondents' Median Salaries	$22,187	$18,019	$20,197	$22,910
Population Median Incomes	$13,710	$20,291	$24,702	$28,964

Note. The data on the general population are from *Money Income of Households, Families, and Persons in the United States: 1982* by E. J. Welniak and M. F. Henson, 1984, Washington, DC: Bureau of the Census. Copyright 1984 by Bureau of the Census. Adapted by permission.

Disregarding the very small group (47) with no college education, the general pattern is that average salaries increase with higher levels of educational attainment. This conclusion is most obvious at the doctoral level—95.6% of those with PhDs earn above the near-median level.

The question now arises whether hearing-impaired professional or managerial workers are rewarded as well as similarly educated workers in the general population. Table 24 compares the median salaries of the hearing-impaired respondents with the normally hearing population over 25.

The low median income for the general population with a high school education or less is to be expected since the general population data cover all occupations. Such coverage being the case, the higher medians shown for the general population over the hearing-impaired professionals and managers indicate that the respondents earn less, on the whole, than similarly educated workers in the general population.

Summary

Most of the hearing-impaired professionals who participated in the survey obtained their basic training through education. The survey examined their education beginning with high school graduation. More than half of the respondents graduated from residential schools for hearing-impaired students. Historically, these schools have attracted a majority of the early and the more severely hearing impaired. Most of the respondents who were less severely hearing impaired and those deafened after age 12 went to general public high schools. About one third of the respondents fell in this category.

The respondents who attended general colleges had access to a number of support services. Notetakers and interpreters were the most available services. The respondents majored in a variety of subjects; however, the most frequently cited majors were education, English, mathematics, business, and psychology.

In comparison with professional/managerial peers in the general population, the hearing-impaired respondents were much more highly educated—92.7% had college degrees whereas only 51.8% of the comparable general population group had such degrees. However, the respondents' median salary was less than median money income of the general population at every education level.

Chapter Four
JOB FINDING METHODS

Terry H. Coye

Typically, labor market studies investigating the status attainment of workers focus on two areas. The first area includes the characteristics of the workers (e.g., family background and education); the second area includes the characteristics of the job market (e.g., openness and salary ranges available).

Both Crammatte (1968; present volume) and Schroedel (1976/1977) have explored these two areas in depth. Between the two areas, however, is a third area which has become the object of more careful study in recent years and which is the subject of this chapter: job finding methods. Job finding method refers to any means by which a job seeker hears about a job opportunity. A tip from a friend, an advertisement in a newspaper, and a listing at an employment agency are all examples of job finding methods.

Occasionally the job finds the worker, as in the case of a lecturer offered a job by an audience member who is impressed with the lecturer's presentation. Much more often, however, the unemployed or

The author appreciates the help of Shari Barnartt, Vicki Freimuth, and John Schroedel in reviewing the drafts of this chapter and the assistance and encouragement given by Alan Crammatte and Susan King in bringing the project to completion.

dissatisfied worker initiates and conducts the search for leads to job opportunities.

Job finding data on blue-collar workers have been collected by labor economists since the 1930s. Interest in job finding methods in these studies grew from a desire to measure the effects of universal techniques (e.g., the use of an employment agency or a national job advertisement) to neutralize the constraints that family background and region placed on the occupational choices of the worker (Granovetter, 1974; Sjoberg, 1960). Therefore, job finding methods were categorized as either *formal methods* (employment agencies and advertisements) or *informal methods* (any other method that did not make use of a disinterested intermediary) (Granovetter, 1974; Rees & Shultz, 1970; Reid, 1972; Stumpf & Collarelli, 1980). In virtually all of the blue-collar studies, the great majority of workers secured their jobs through informal methods; relatively few used formal methods (De Schweinetz, 1932; Lester, 1954; Lurie & Rayack, 1968; Sheppard & Belitsky, 1966; Ullman & Taylor, 1965).

Studies of white-collar workers, though fewer in number than studies of blue-collar workers, have shown similar results (Brown, 1965; Shapero, Howell, & Tombaugh, 1965; Shultz, 1962). The actual percentages of use of advertisements and agencies vary from study to study and group to group, but all studies have shown that a majority of white-collar workers used informal methods to find their jobs.

In general, studies have demonstrated that workers who used informal methods had more positive labor market outcomes than workers who used formal methods. Reid (1972), for example, found that displaced British blue-collar workers who used informal methods tended to find new jobs more quickly and to be more satisfied with those jobs than their compatriots who used formal methods. McKersie and Ullman's study (1966) of Harvard alumni and Gutteridge's study (1971) of business school graduates found that respondents who used informal methods earned more than respondents who used formal methods.

In 1974, Mark S. Granovetter published the results of his study of the job finding methods of professional, technical, and managerial workers in Newton, Massachusetts. His study is significant first of all because he divided informal methods into two separate categories: *personal contacts* and *direct application*. Personal contacts includes the friends, relatives, and acquaintances who provide information about job openings; direct application refers to the practice of finding a job by simply sending a resume to a company or walking in the front door and filling out a job application without knowing if an appropriate job is available.

This separation allowed Granovetter to investigate the nature and use of contacts as conduits for job information. He found that personal contacts still accounted for more than half of all jobs found by his sample. Direct application and formal means each accounted for less than 20% of all jobs found (Granovetter, 1974).

Granovetter's study is also significant because it indicated that workers who found their jobs through personal contacts, rather than through more informal methods, were more likely to secure better jobs and to be more satisfied with their jobs than workers who used any other method. He concluded that job seekers who use personal contacts (i.e., those who get job leads through their network of friends, relatives, and acquaintances) are able to locate more job openings and are able to get more information about each potential job than those who do not use contacts.

Studies conducted since Granovetter's have continued to show that using personal contacts is a popular job finding method (Langlois, 1977; Lin, Ensel, & Vaughn, 1981). However, a study of two-year college graduates by Allen and Keaveny (1980) found that most of these graduates used formal methods instead of personal contacts. Furthermore, salary was not found to be significantly related to method used, and occupational levels, when found to be significantly related to method, tended to be higher among respondents who had used formal methods.

Allen and Keaveny suggested that the differences between their findings and Granovetter's might be attributed to the differences in the ages of their respondents. Their respondents were younger and, therefore, may not have had networks as well developed as those of Granovetter's respondents.

Allen and Keaveny also suggested that labor markets for the engineering and business students they studied may have been tight, which caused employers to become more aggressive in using formal methods such as on-campus visits to recruit new employees. Under these circumstances, it was perhaps easier for job seekers to find several good jobs through formal means rather than through contacts (Allen & Keaveny, pp. 981–982).

THE INFLUENCE OF NETWORKS

In the last decade, the importance of informal job finding methods has aroused the curiosity of sociologists and communication scientists. If friends and relatives are more important resources than advertisements and employment agencies for getting job leads, then an individual's network of personal contacts forms an important link between the potential worker and the job opening. The network, however, is also an important constraint in the labor market. This happens because the leads an individual gets through informal channels are limited to whatever job openings his or her personal contacts know about.

The methods that hearing workers use to find jobs appear to have important effects on their occupational status attainment. It therefore becomes important to ask if this is as true for hearing-impaired workers. The question, Do hearing-impaired job seekers have a network to help them find jobs?, also is important to this study. Croneberg (1976) suggested that

> everywhere in North America, there are deaf people using sign language who are part of a network of social contacts. . . . The deaf as a group have social ties with each other that extend farther across the nation than similarities of perhaps any other American minority group. (p. 310)

Higgins (1980), in his study of the deaf community as an outsider community, claimed that through "various avenues of association, deaf people can keep in contact with each other in ever widening circles. First at the local level and gradually building to the national level, a network of relationships among deaf people is established" (p. 75). Not only does this national network create a "sense of solidarity" (p. 75) among deaf people, Higgins added, but it also serves as a medium for the transfer of information: "Newsworthy events within the deaf community are likely to become common knowledge not only within that community, but also throughout the country" (p. 73).

In order to discover whether this network also provides information about job openings to hearing-impaired job seekers, the study reported here was conducted. It addressed the following questions:
1. What methods do hearing-impaired professionals use to find the jobs they hold?
2. What are the effects, if any, of the job finding method selected on the salary and job satisfaction of hearing-impaired professionals?
3. Is there any evidence of a network that provides job information to hearing-impaired job seekers?

THE SURVEY

Crammatte began receiving responses to his professional employment questionnaire in the fall of 1983. At that time, it was decided that additional questionnaires should be sent to the respondents to collect information about the methods they used to find their jobs.

In preparing the second questionnaire, certain questions were included so that the results could be compared to surveys of hearing professional workers. Of all the available studies of job finding methods, only Granovetter's (1974) focused on a population of hearing workers with characteristics similar to those of the hearing-impaired population under study by Crammatte. Granovetter collected data from 300 randomly selected white-collar workers (200 through personal interview, 100 through mail survey) in the greater Boston area. The population of hearing workers in professional, technical, and managerial jobs he targeted was quite similar to the hearing-impaired population under study here. Several of Granovetter's mail survey questions were included on the questionnaire sent to hearing-impaired professionals so that the results could be compared.

Because funds for the job finding study were limited, only half of the respondents to the Professional Employment Questionnaire received the second questionnaire. The recipients were randomly selected from Crammatte's mailing list (see Appendix A) of appropriate respondents. Eventually, Crammatte received 1735 usable responses; of these, one half (or 867) received the job finding questionnaire.

Twenty-three of the mailed questionnaires were undeliverable because of inadequate addresses. A total of 739 responses were received;

however, 13 of these responses were invalid because they were received from subjects who had not been selected from Crammatte's list to receive a second questionnaire. This puzzling result may have been due to Crammatte's snowball data collection technique, which asked hearing-impaired professionals to pass on information and names of other hearing-impaired professionals. It is possible that some respondents did not have time to answer the second questionnaire, so they passed it along to a friend who did. Five of the 13 unsolicited responses came from hearing-impaired spouses of intended respondents. All 13 invalid responses were excluded from data analysis.

A total of 726 valid responses, then, were received out of the potential pool of 867 responses (a response rate of 83.7%). Though this rate is exceptionally high for a mail survey, it is not surprising when one considers that the entire sample was selected from a pool of persons who had already responded to a similar questionnaire.

Twenty-two (or 3.0%) of the 726 valid responses were also excluded from data analysis, for the following reasons: 3 responses were illegible, 5 responses were returned blank (with letters attached), and 14 responses were from professionals who had been promoted to their current positions from lower positions within the organization. (Since the purpose of this study was to investigate how job seekers find leads to new jobs in new organizations, data from promoted workers would not be enlightening.) The total maximum number of usable responses, therefore, was 706.

Survey Method Problems

Two biases resulted from the methods used in this survey. The first bias resulted from the exclusive use of a mail survey to collect data. If time and money had permitted the use of personal interviews, follow-up questions could have probed the job finding process more deeply and clarified inconsistent responses. For example, a few respondents who initially indicated that they found out about their jobs through direct application mentioned, in incidental comments elsewhere on the questionnaire, that they had used another method as well. Deeper probing would be necessary to clarify exactly which method had been used first. Since explanatory comments were not required of all respondents, some incorrect responses may appear in the data. It is assumed that any incorrect responses that do appear are randomly distributed, however, and do not seriously affect the results.

Another bias inherent in the survey resulted from the exclusive use of data from employees. Some employers may constrain the range of usable job finding methods by refusing to accept direct applications, for example, or by only hiring individuals known personally to themselves or their associates. In cases such as these, employers predetermine the job finding methods that job seekers must use to secure employment.

Though not a bias in the study, an additional constraint on the interpretation of results arose from the definition of *job finding method*. As used here, the term refers to any means by which a respondent first heard about the job he or she had found, accepted, and held at the time the questionnaire was received. It does not include those methods job seekers used before or after they found out about the job they eventually took. For example, a job seeker may have found 10 jobs by using personal contacts, but decided to take the one job listed with an employment agency. The data collected would include only the latter method.

SURVEY RESULTS

Question 1.

What Methods Did Hearing-Impaired Professionals Use to Find the Jobs They Hold?

Getting job leads from personal contacts was by far the most often used job finding method. This method was used successfully by more than half of all respondents to the survey (358 respondents, or 51.0% of the sample), which means that the personal contacts method was used more often than all other methods combined (see Table 25).

As Table 26 indicates, the vast majority (316, or 88.3%) of personal contacts were friends and acquaintances. The contacts developed while respondents were completing an internship, a student teaching assignment, or other short-term employment, plus those from relatives and family friends, accounted for less than 12% of all contacts used.

Table 25
Job Finding Methods Used By Hearing-Impaired Professionals

Job Finding Method	Hearing-Impaired Professionals	
	Number	Percent
Formal Means	159	22.7
Personal Contact	358	51.0
Direct Application	112	16.0
Other	68	9.7
No Response	4	.6
Total	701	100.0

The second most popular job finding method was the use of formal means, (i.e., the use of formal intermediaries—people or media—whose primary function is to connect workers and employers). This method can include the use of employment agencies, job advertisements, vocational rehabilitation counselors, placement offices, etc., which are the means of finding jobs that are most commonly associated with a job search.

Though one out of every four hearing-impaired professionals in the sample found their jobs through formal means, this method represented a distant second to the use of personal contacts. More than twice as many respondents used friends, relatives, or acquaintances as used employment agencies and newspaper classified ads.

The most often used formal means technique was the posted or published job advertisement, which led to jobs for more than one third of the respondents who used formal means. Nearly as many re-

Table 26
Subcategories of Personal Contacts Used by
Hearing-Impaired Professionals

Subcategory	Hearing-Impaired Professionals	
	Number	Percent
Friends and acquaintances	316	88.3
Relatives and family friends	17	4.7
Internships, student teaching, etc.	25	7.0
Total	358	100.0

spondents secured job leads from college placement offices, whereas employment agencies and vocational rehabilitation offices combined found jobs for only one fifth of the respondents who used formal means. The remaining respondents used "other formal means," which included finding job leads through conventions, career days, recruiter visits, or by assignment (e.g., a minister was assigned to a new parish by a bishop).

Table 27 shows that hearing-impaired professionals made greater use of college placement offices than employment agencies or vocational rehabilitation services. Given the number of agencies that specialize in executive, managerial, and technical job placement, one would expect hearing-impaired professionals to make greater use of this type of formal means. Either employment agencies are not very helpful to deaf people seeking professional jobs, or deaf professionals do not seek them out.

Only 16.0 percent (112) of the respondents to this survey found their current job through direct application (sending a resume to a company or contacting the company without knowing first if any jobs are available). Although a distant third among the job methods used, the respondents who used this method displayed the most patience and industry of all job seekers in the sample. One respondent moved to a new city simply because he had always wanted to live in that part of the country. He had no job or job leads there, but he did have skill as a bookkeeper for a grocery store. His job search consisted of opening the yellow pages to a list of grocery stores and contacting each in order until he found an opening. Another respondent, a chemical engineer,

Table 27
Subcategories of Formal Means Used by
Hearing-Impaired Professionals

Subcategory	Hearing-Impaired Professionals	
	Number	Percent
Published or posted job advertisement	57	35.8
College placement office	53	33.3
Employment agency or vocational rehabilitation	33	20.8
Other formal means	16	10.1
Total	159	100.0

first saw the name of the chemical firm he later joined on the side of a company truck that happened to pass him on the street.

The category called *other* is a composite category that includes those methods which are not one of the other three. For example, 7 (10.3%) of the workers in this category created their own jobs; 15 (22.1%) were self-employed. Because of the small number of cases in this category (68, or 9.7% of the total sample), further discussion will focus only on the three larger categories of job finding methods—formal means, personal contacts and direct application.

Comparison of the Job Finding Methods of Hearing and Hearing-Impaired Professionals

Granovetter's sample (1974) differs from the hearing-impaired sample in three important ways: his sample included, presumably, only hearing people; he collected information only from men; and his sample included only workers who had held their current jobs for 5 years or less. In order to compare the results from the hearing-impaired sample with Granovetter's, a matching subgroup of hearing-impaired men who had held their jobs for 5 years or less was selected. A comparison of the job finding methods of Granovetter's sample, the hearing-impaired subgroup, and the whole hearing-impaired group appears in Table 28.

Table 28
Job Finding Methods Used by Professional Groups
(In %)

	Professional Groups		
Method Used	Hearing Professionals [a] n=258	Hearing-Impaired Professionals (Comparable Group) n=203	Hearing-Impaired Professionals (Total Sample) n=697
Formal Means	18.8	27.2	22.8
Personal Contact	55.7	49.0	51.3
Direct Application	18.8	13.6	16.1
Other	6.7	10.2	9.8

[a] The data in column 1 are from *Getting a Job: A Study of Contacts and Careers* (p. 11) by M. S. Granovetter, 1974, Cambridge: Harvard University Press. Adapted by permission.

The results of the current study and Granovetter's study are similar in two important ways. First, about half of each group used personal contacts to find their current jobs. This method outstrips any other method by many percentage points in all groups. Like their hearing counterparts, more hearing-impaired professionals heard about the jobs they eventually took through friends and relatives than through any other method. Second, formal means and direct application accounted for many of the remaining cases. The "other" category, which includes any method that is not one of the first three, is quite small. Formal means, personal contacts and direct application, as defined by both studies, successfully account for nearly all means of finding jobs used by both populations.

Granovetter found no differences in the degree of formal means and direct application his respondents used; each of the two categories accounted for 18.8% of the total. Within the comparable subgroup of hearing-impaired professionals, however, formal means were used twice as often as direct application. Though not the most important method of finding jobs for either group, formal means seem to be used much more frequently by hearing-impaired professionals than by their hearing counterparts.

Question 2.

What are the Effects, If Any, of the Job Finding Method Used on the Salary and Job Satisfaction of Hearing-Impaired Professionals?

Salary and Job Finding Method

Granovetter found that the use of personal contacts led more often to better paying jobs. Nearly half (45.5%) of the hearing workers who used personal contacts secured higher paying jobs, whereas only 30% (less than one third) of those using formal means and 19.2% (less than one fifth) of those using direct application found higher paying jobs (1974, p. 14).

When salary was cross-tabulated by job finding method for the comparable subgroup of hearing-impaired workers, however, no significant results were obtained (chi-square = 4.29413, df = 3, p = .2314). For hearing-impaired workers, no job finding method was statistically more likely than any other to lead to a higher paying job.

Job Satisfaction and Job Finding Method

Means of collecting data on job satisfaction were slightly different in the present survey than in Granovetter's. Granovetter asked respondents to indicate their overall level of job satisfaction by selecting *very satisfied, fairly satisfied, neither satisfied nor dissatisfied, fairly dissatisfied,* or *very dissatisfied.* The questionnaire sent to hearing-impaired professionals asked respondents to answer six separate questions related to job satisfaction. On a four-point scale (*like very much, like a little, dislike a little,* and *dislike very much*) respondents ranked how much they liked their (a) salaries, (b) supervisors, (c) kind of work, (d) chances for promotion (if appropriate), (e) co-workers, and (f) those who worked under them. When cross-tabulated by job finding method, significant results for the comparable subgroup of hearing-impaired professionals were found only on the first three measures (for the last three measures, respectively, chi-square = 3.14313, $df = 3$, $p = .3701$; chi-square = 5.28971, $df = 3$, $p = .1518$; and chi-square = 1.69161, $df = 3$, $p = .6388$).

Granovetter found that hearing professionals who used personal contacts to find their jobs were most likely to express high satisfaction with their jobs (although the difference between results for personal contacts and direct application was very small). More than half (54.2%) of hearing professionals who used personal contacts reported that they were very satisfied with their jobs, whereas a slightly lower percentage (52.8%) of those who used direct application, and a much lower percentage (30.0%) of those who used formal means, were very satisfied with their jobs (1974, p. 13).

Among hearing-impaired professionals, however, those who used "other" or formal means to find their jobs were most likely to express strong liking of their supervisors and kind of work (see Tables 29 and 30). Considering that many individuals in this category came by their jobs in particularly unusual ways (by creating their own jobs or becoming self-employed, for example), it is not surprising that they showed great job satisfaction.

It is surprising that those among Granovetter's respondents who used "other" methods did not show greater satisfaction. Because of the composite nature of the category and the extremely small number of cases that constitute it, interpretation of the results of the "other"

Table 29
Relation of Respondents' Liking of Supervisors to
Their Job Finding Method
(In %)

	Job Finding Method			
Level of Liking	Formal Means $n=59$	Personal Contacts $n=105$	Direct Application $n=28$	Other $n=16$
Like very much	72.9	56.2	46.4	81.2
Like less than very much	27.1	43.8	53.6	18.8

Note. Chi-square = 9.80347; df = 3; p = .0203; missing observations = 27.

Table 30
Relation of Respondents' Liking of Kind of Work to
Their Job Finding Method
(In %)

	Job Finding Method			
Level of Liking	Formal Means $n=62$	Personal Contacts $n=116$	Direct Application $n=30$	Other $n=24$
Like very much	77.4	75.0	56.7	91.7
Like less than very much	22.6	25.0	43.3	8.3

Note. Chi-square = 9.12688; df = 3; p = .0277; missing observations = 3.

category must be limited and cautious; only one or two more cases added to the category could radically alter the results.

Question 3.

Is There Any Evidence of a Network That Provides Job Information to Hearing-Impaired Professionals?

Direct observation of a network is not possible using a mail survey like the present one because it gathered data from only one part of the network. The smallest single unit of any network is the link between two individuals (Rogers & Kincaid, 1981). In order to observe the transfer of information to the job seeker through a link with a personal contact, it would be necessary to gather data from both individuals.

In order to observe an extended network, it would be necessary to gather data from all individuals included. However, it is possible to infer the operation of a network from the data collected in the present survey by looking at the relationships among the job finding method used, the sector of the job, the kind of job secured, and the communication preference of the job seeker.

Kinds of Jobs and Networks

Individuals within a network will tend to have the same information (Granovetter, 1973). Therefore, job information from personal contacts in a network will tend to lead the job seeker to the same kinds of jobs. Two indicators of kind of job appear in the data: *job sector* and *type of employer*.

Sectors and Job Finding Methods

Important differences in the use of job finding methods appear when hearing-impaired professionals are divided according to whether their jobs are in the *deaf sector* or the *hearing sector*. Deaf sector jobs are those which directly serve hearing-impaired people or which employ deaf people because of their hearing status (such as the National Theatre of the Deaf); hearing sector jobs are those which serve the general public (see p. 74 in chap. 5).

As Table 31 indicates, personal contact was the most often used job finding method for both sectors. The two sectors differ significantly, however, in their relative use of personal contacts and formal means. Personal contacts were used more often to find deaf sector jobs than to find hearing sector jobs, whereas formal means were used more often to find hearing sector jobs than deaf sector jobs.

The results represented in Table 31 may be explained by the existence of a network that assisted deaf professionals in finding jobs in the deaf sector. One would expect that deaf professionals would have more contacts—a more extensive network—among other persons working in the deaf sector than among those working in the hearing sector. There are, after all, more people like themselves (e.g., who are hearing-impaired, use signs, or graduated from schools for the deaf) in the deaf sector than in the hearing sector. The respondents' friends,

Table 31
Job Finding Methods Used in Different Job Sectors
(In %)

Job Finding Method	Job Sector	
	Deaf Sector $n=510$	Hearing Sector $n=185$
Formal Means	18.8	34.1
Personal Contact	55.1	41.5
Direct Application	16.5	14.1
Other	9.6	10.3

Note. Chi-square = 19.11310; df = 3; p = .0003; missing observations = 6.

both at work and socially, are more likely to be deaf and to work in the deaf sector, so information from their network of friends is more likely to be effective in finding deaf sector jobs.

One would also expect, however, that the network would not be as extensive in the hearing sector and that personal contacts would be a less useful job finding method for that sector. Therefore, hearing-impaired workers seeking jobs in the hearing sector must rely more heavily on the assistance of impersonal intermediaries (formal means).

One problem with the interpretation of Table 31, however, appears in the results for direct application. If impersonal methods tended to be used when personal contacts were not effective, one would expect that direct application would have been used by a greater percentage of hearing sector job holders than of deaf sector job holders. This was not the case; though results were close, direct application was used by a slightly larger percentage of deaf sector workers than of hearing sector workers.

One possible explanation is that workers may have applied directly to contacts. Incidental comments by some respondents who used direct application indicated that they knew the employer before they applied for the job, even though they did not find out about the job before they filled out the application form. Typical of these responses is the case of an accountant who had worked briefly for an accounting firm in his hometown after graduating from college. He found a better job in another state and moved away, but returned several years later to care for a disabled parent. Not knowing if any jobs were available, he went to his old employer and applied for any openings that might be had. The employer remembered his past work and hired him on the spot.

The questionnaires never asked respondents directly to discuss this kind of job finding process. If many other respondents who used direct application were like the accountant, it would be easy to see that personal contacts are an important element in direct application and that the two methods are more similar than they appear. Unfortunately, we have no way of firmly establishing this connection from the data collected.

Another explanation of these results appears when job sector, job finding method, and selected characteristics of the worker are considered simultaneously. Before discussing this second explanation, however, the relationships between network access and job finding method must be explored further.

Networks: Job Finding Methods and the Deaf Community

Hearing-impaired professionals who use personal contacts to find jobs were the group most likely to find deaf sector jobs. However, many others in the sample did not use personal contacts to find deaf sector jobs, and many were not employed in the deaf sector at all. If a network that reached inside the deaf sector provided information about job openings for some respondents, it apparently did not for others. These others may have been outside of the network and therefore unable to tap its resources.

Not all hearing-impaired people, needless to say, associate to any great degree with other hearing-impaired people. They are deaf, but outside the deaf community; their personal contacts would not necessarily have any more information about deaf sector jobs than those of most hearing people.

Respondents were not asked if they were members of the deaf community, and it is unlikely that clear answers to such questions could be made. Researchers disagree on appropriate indicators of boundaries between deaf and hearing communities. Linguists have tended to view the deaf community as a language community that uses American Sign Language (Markowicz & Woodward, 1978; Padden & Markowicz, 1975). Nash and Nash (1981) claim that the use of signs alone is a sufficient boundary indicator. Higgins, however, claims that "signing is not a sufficient condition, though it is a necessary condition for membership in deaf communities" (1980, p. 68). He suggests that three factors are important to attaining membership: identification with deaf people, shared experiences with deaf people, and participation in deaf community activities (1980, p. 38).

However, the concern in the present study lies less with community membership than with the kinds of networks to which a job seeker has access. The use or non-use of signs as a medium of communication may not be a sufficient condition for membership in the deaf community, but certainly it designates a clear boundary between networks. A network in which information is transferred through signs will be limited to individuals who can sign; a network in which information is transferred through speech will be limited to individuals who can speak. Bridges between signing and speaking networks are possible, of course, since some individuals can both speak and sign with equal fluency. However, most individuals have a preference for one method of communication or the other.

In the present study, respondents were asked to indicate their preferred method of communication by selecting *sign language, speaking/lipreading, writing*, or *other method*. As Table 32 indicates, more than half of the respondents (399, or 56.9%) preferred using sign language. A much smaller number of respondents (112, or 16%) preferred speech/speechreading and very few (6, or .9%) preferred writing. A surprisingly large group of respondents (120, or 23.8%) selected the other method category for varying reasons.

Some of the respondents wrote on the questionnaire that they preferred to communicate using both signs and speech/speechreading (or lip movements) at the same time (i.e., simultaneous communication). Others indicated that they were equally comfortable using any method of communication. Some respondents wrote in *total communication*, which might have referred to either the simultaneous use of signs and speech/speechreading, or the use of whatever method is appropriate to each communication situation. Others did not state any clear preference.

Since the purpose of the questionnaire was to investigate the differences between networks available to signers and speakers, the responses to this question were reduced to three categories: sign language, speech/speechreading, and other (which included writing).

Table 32
Distribution of Preferred Methods of Communication

Method	Respondents Number	Percent
Speech/speechreading	112	16.0
Sign language	399	56.9
Writing	6	.9
Other		
Simultaneous communication	33	4.7
Total communication	41	5.8
Preference not clear	93	13.3
No Response	17	2.4
Total	701	100.0

Job finding method was cross-tabulated by preferred method of communication to determine if signers used different methods to find jobs than did speakers. As Table 33 indicates, all three groups used personal contacts more than any other method. However, speakers were the most likely group to use formal means and/or direct application. Signers and others were more likely than speakers to use personal contacts.

This difference could be explained by the effects of a signing network. Information about jobs that are available to and desired by signers is passed around a network of signers. It is logical to conclude that signers use personal contacts more than other modes because they have more contacts who have appropriate job information. Speakers,

Table 33
Relation of Job Finding Method to Preferred Method of Communication
(In %)

Job Finding Method	Preferred Method of Communication		
	Speech/Speechreading $n=112$	Sign Language $n=398$	Other $n=171$
Formal Means	33.0	23.1	15.2
Personal Contacts	34.8	55.3	57.3
Direct Application	18.8	14.1	15.8
Other	13.4	7.5	11.7

Note. Chi-square = 23.06264; df = 6; p = .0008; missing observations = 20.

who generally do not have access to this information, have to rely more heavily on formal means and direct application. Interestingly, workers in the "other" category were even more likely to have used personal contacts than signers; they were also the least likely of all groups to have used formal means. If it is correct to assume that high use of personal contacts indicates access to network information, then "other" workers may have had access to both signing and speaking networks.

But what kind of information is available from signing and from speaking networks? A clearer picture of network operation can be drawn when data on job finding method, preferred method of communication, and job sector are considered simultaneously.

Job Sector, Job Finding Method, and Networks

The results obtained from the questionnaire indicate that there is a relationship between networks and job sectors. Apparently, the network available to signers provided them with more usable information about deaf sector jobs, while the network available to speakers provided them with more usable information about hearing sector jobs. As Table 34 indicates, in the deaf sector, signers were more likely to use personal contacts than were speakers. In the hearing sector, these results were reversed; speakers were more likely than signers to use personal contacts.

Table 34
Job Sector Analysis of Job Finding Method by
Preferred Method of Communication
(In %)

	Preferred Method of Communication					
	Deaf Sector			*Hearing Sector*		
Job Finding Method	*Speech/ Speechreading* $n=60$	*Sign Language* $n=313$	*Other* $n=124$	*Speech/ Speechreading* $n=52$	*Sign Language* $n=85$	*Other* $n=45$
Formal Means	31.7	19.5	12.1	34.6	36.4	24.4
Personal Contacts	26.7	61.0	58.1	44.2	34.1	57.9
Direct Application	28.3	11.8	18.5	7.7	22.4	4.4
Other	13.3	7.7	11.3	13.5	7.1	13.3

Note. For the deaf sector, chi-square = 31.20034, df = 6, p = .0001; for the hearing sector, chi-square = 15.77825, df = 6, p = .015; missing observations = 22.

Table 34 also shows that relative use of formal means and direct application by signers and speakers also reversed between sectors. Speakers were more likely than signers to use direct application and formal means to find deaf sector jobs, whereas signers were more likely to use them to find hearing sector jobs.

Results for formal means and direct application may be related to lack of access to a usable network. If job seekers had easy access to job information from their networks, they used them; if their networks did not have sufficient information, job seekers had to rely more heavily on other means. Speakers had less access to usable network information about deaf sector jobs because this information was more prevalent in signing networks. Therefore, speakers were more likely than signers to turn to formal means and direct application to find deaf sector jobs. Signing networks were similarly less helpful in finding hearing sector jobs, so signers turned to other means to find hearing sector jobs.

If these speculations are correct, the results for workers in the "other" categories in Table 34 suggest that these workers have access to networks that are useful in finding jobs in either sector. In both sectors, approximately 58% of "other" workers used personal contacts to find their jobs. In the hearing sector, in fact, workers in the "other" category were the most likely group to have used personal contacts. "Other" workers may have made greater use of personal contacts because information from signing networks may have led to different jobs in the hearing sector than information from speaking networks. Since "other" workers had access to both kinds of networks, they may have had more usable information than either signers or speakers.

Limitations of Networks: Type of Employer and Job Finding Methods

According to the responses received on the questionnaire, networks appear to be relatively less effective in finding jobs with certain categories of employers (see Table 35). As Table 35 indicates, more respondents in every category of employment found their jobs through personal contacts. The largest percentage of respondents using personal contacts to obtain jobs (56.0%) were those who worked in educational institutions.

Table 35
Breakdown of Job Finding Method By Type of Employer
(In %)

Job Finding Method	Private Business n=110	Educational Institution n=411	Government n=132	Other n=36
Formal Means	33.6	16.5	34.8	19.4
Personal Contact	43.6	56.0	47.1	33.3
Direct Application	15.5	18.7	9.8	11.1
Other	7.3	8.8	8.3	36.2

Note. Chi-square = 59.19497; df = 9; p = .0001; missing observations = 12.

The largest differences between types of employers in Table 35 appear in the second and third most used job finding methods for each category. For private business and government, formal means was the second most often used method, with the difference between personal contacts and formal means less than 13% in each category. Direct application was a distant third for these two types of employers. For jobs in educational institutions, however, direct application (18.7%) was a very distant second, with formal means (16.5%) only slightly behind.

Job holders working in educational institutions were the group most likely to have used direct application (18.7%), though the percentage of workers in private business who used direct application was nearly as large (15.5%). The percentage of workers in educational institutions who used formal means (16.5%), however, was less than half that of workers in private business (33.6%) or in government (34.8%).

In sum, hearing-impaired professionals employed by any of the four types of employers were more likely to have used personal contacts than any other job finding method. However, workers in educational institutions were more likely than other workers to have used personal contacts and direct application, whereas workers in government and private business were more likely to have used formal means.

In order to determine if signers tended to become employed by different kinds of employers than speakers, type of employer was

Table 36
Preferred Method of Communication Used in Different Employment Settings

	Preferred Method of Communication		
Type of Employer	Speech/ Speechreading n=112	Sign Language n=393	Other n=171
Private Business	25.0	12.0	19.3
Educational Institution	53.6	63.3	54.3
Government	14.3	20.1	21.1
Other	7.1	4.6	5.3

Note. Chi-square = 16.21805; df = 6; p = .0126; missing observations = 25.

cross-tabulated with preferred method of communication. As Table 36 shows, educational institutions were the biggest employers of all workers, employing more than half of all hearing-impaired professionals. Signers were the group most likely to be employed in educational institutions, whereas speakers were the group most likely to be employed in private business. Signers and others were more likely than speakers to be employed by government.

To determine if job finding methods could account for the results in Table 36, cross-tabulations of job finding method and preferred method of communication were run, controlling for type of employer. Only the results for workers in educational institutions were found to be statistically significant (for private business, chi-square = 7.98606, df = 6, p = .2391; for government, chi-square = 7.45099, df = 6, p = .2811; for other, chi-square = 7.91311, df = 6, p = .2445).

As Table 37 indicates, workers in educational institutions had used personal contacts more often than any other job finding method. Signers in educational institutions were the group most likely to have used personal contacts, and they were twice as likely to use this method as speakers. Speakers were the group most likely to have used formal means and direct application.

The results shown in Table 37 for workers in educational institutions were similar to the results for all workers in the deaf sector (see Table 34), probably because nearly all jobs (97.1%) held by hearing-impaired professionals in educational institutions were in the deaf sector.

Table 37
Job Finding Methods and Preferred Methods of Communication
Used by Workers in Educational Institutions
(In %)

Job Finding Method	Preferred Method of Communication		
	Speech/ Speechreading $n=60$	Sign Language $n=248$	Other $n=92$
Formal Means	28.3	18.1	5.4
Personal Contacts	31.7	62.1	57.6
Direct Application	26.7	13.3	26.1
Other	13.3	6.5	10.9

Note. Chi-square = 32.29771; $df = 6$; $p = .0001$.

To determine if sector could account for the results in Tables 36 and 37, cross-tabulations of job finding method and job sector were created for each of the categories of employing institutions. No significant results were obtained (for private business, chi-square = 1.98615, $df = 3$, $p = .5753$; for educational institutions, chi-square = 1.5727, $df = 3$, $p = .7633$; for government, chi-square = 5.19198, $df = 3$, $p = .1583$; for other, chi-square = 7.14657, $df = 3$, $p = .0674$).

The lack of significant results in the cross-tabulations reported here suggests that the means of finding jobs among the four types of employers were fairly stable. These methods did not vary greatly by preferred method of communication or by sector. The results reported in the discussion of Table 35 hold true for both signers and speakers and for jobs in both the deaf and hearing sectors. This stability implies that the pathways into jobs with certain types of employers are fairly set; the pathways appear to have more to do with the job than with the preferences of the job seeker.

If networks that help hearing-impaired professionals find jobs exist, they function least well in private business, where only 43.6% (see Table 35) of the jobs were found through personal contacts. In contrast, 56.0% of the respondents who work in educational institutions found their jobs this way.

There appears to be a barrier of some kind that has prevented the respondents to the survey from establishing and/or using personal contacts to secure employment in private businesses. Some possible reasons for this barrier may include the following:

1. Perhaps the businesses represented rely heavily on employment agencies or other formal means and are therefore resistant to blind applications or word-of-mouth recruiting practices.
2. Perhaps the number of deaf people with appropriate skills for a specific job opening in private business are so few and far between that appropriate job lead information is unlikely to reach them.
3. Perhaps discrimination against deaf workers persists most strongly among employers in this category.

Networks appear to have been most effective in finding jobs in educational institutions. One explanation for this is that a relatively small number of institutions train teachers of deaf children. An even smaller number train hearing-impaired teachers, and there are relatively few schools that hire hearing-impaired teachers. The world of education of deaf people is a small one, so a well-established network among school administrators and personnel in teacher preparation programs may be operating as the most important means of matching job openings with available teachers.

Summary

Like their hearing counterparts, hearing-impaired professionals were much more likely to use personal contacts to find jobs than any other job finding method. Men and women, younger workers and older workers, signers and nonsigners, teachers, lawyers, actors and managers, the moderately deaf, the profoundly deaf—all were more likely to have gotten job leads from friends or relatives than through all other methods combined. Apparently "who you know" is as important to deaf professionals as it is to hearing professionals. These results suggest that deaf job seekers should consider their friends and acquaintances as primary sources of job information and essential elements in their job search strategies.

A disturbing finding in this study was the greater use of formal means by hearing-impaired professionals than by their hearing counterparts, especially to secure job leads in the hearing sector. Deaf professionals appear to have had fewer useful contacts in the hearing sector and/or they have encountered greater resistance to their applications in this sector from employers unfamiliar with deaf workers. This resistance has necessitated a greater reliance on a third party (i.e., formal means) to obtain jobs.

The reliance on formal means is disturbing in light of the probable stagnation or even decrease in the growth of deaf sector jobs. The push for mainstreaming handicapped children into traditional public school programs, coupled with the drive to reduce federal social services in recent years, means that deaf job seekers increasingly must look to private business and state and local governments for professional job opportunities. Without useful contacts in the hearing sector and/or influential intermediaries to overcome employer resistance, the hearing-impaired job seeker may find job leads harder to discover and professional employment increasingly elusive. Serious thought needs to be given to finding ways to overcome the disadvantages faced by hearing-impaired persons in finding employment in the hearing sector. One way may be to find out how some hearing-impaired job seekers were able to establish and use contacts in the hearing sector. There may be more than luck involved, and it may be possible to identify specific, replicable techniques that could be taught to others.

A second way may be to look more closely at the formal means that have been successfully employed. More respondents used college placement offices than used employment agencies perhaps because, in addition to providing sources for job openings, these offices actively promote deaf job seekers among potential employers.

More data need to be collected on the information provided and actions taken by others that assisted the job seeker both to find the job and to get hired. Perhaps this information could be used to create employment organizations that could provide services to hearing-impaired job seekers who are not connected to colleges.

On a more positive note, the results in this study provide some evidence that special networks are helping hearing-impaired individuals find jobs. More specific research is needed to determine what these networks are like, who they connect, and what kinds of services and information they provide. To discover this information, several important questions must be answered: Do the networks play a role not only in finding jobs but in helping the job seeker prepare for and actually secure the job? What other kinds of information are present in the networks? Do hearing people play a special role, such as bridging networks of deaf people with other kinds of networks and providing information otherwise not available? Do deaf people equally skilled in signs and speech function as bridges between signing and speaking networks? Are the networks truly national, as Croneberg has suggested? Are networks of deaf people different in any significant way from networks of hearing people? Do these networks play a role in defining and maintaining the deaf community?

The answers to these and similar questions could provide important new insights into the nature of the deaf community in particular and the operation of networks in general.

Chapter Five
WORKING CONDITIONS

A striking finding of this survey is that 1,091 (62.9%) of the respondents reported being employed by educational institutions (see Table 38). This preponderance of respondents in the field of education raises numerous questions: Why does such a large proportion of our top talent choose education of deaf children (only 4 of the 1,091 are employed as public school teachers)? Are aspects of the respondents' hearing impairments determining factors in career choice? Does working with or for hearing-impaired persons provide more or less job satisfaction? What, in general, is the difference between serving deaf people and serving the general public?

To seek answers to such questions, the concept of a dual labor market will be used. Studies of the work force and labor markets in recent years have given considerable attention to dual (segmented) labor markets. The segmentation has been between career-type employment and intermittent, unskilled labor (Rosenberg, 1981). Such extreme job differentiation obviously does not exist among professional workers. Nevertheless, there does seem to be a duality in the labor market for professional workers with hearing impairments. This duality rests upon the question of whom the workers serve.

In this study, the two labor market sectors (hearing and deaf) were determined by clientele. Workers in the deaf sector serve hearing-impaired clients or are in occupations in which their disability is not a hindrance. Examples of these occupations include teaching hearing-impaired students, counseling hearing-impaired clients, ministering to a deaf congregation, acting, and coordinating or providing sign language instruction.

In the hearing sector there are no special clients; sign language skills are of little or no use; and the working environment is oral. The deaf sector is characterized by provision of human services, ease of communication, ready entry, stable employment, and lower salaries. The hearing sector, which consists mostly of government and corporate employers, is characterized by difficult entry, communication problems, higher salaries, and, possibly, greater mobility.

Those 1,072 professionals employed in schools for deaf pupils are not only a majority of all respondents; they also represent 80.5% of the workers in the deaf sector. The next highest group of deaf sector workers (9.9%) is employed by government agencies, and many of these respondents are rehabilitation counselors. In the hearing sector, government and private business employ the great majority of hearing-impaired professional workers (44.1% and 43.0%, respectively).

Table 38
Labor Market Sector of Current Employer

Current Employer	Deaf Sector Number of Respondents	Percent	Hearing Sector Number of Respondents	Percent	Total (Both Sectors) Number	Percent
Private Business	76	5.7	173	43.0	249	14.4
Self-Employed	14	1.1	26	6.5	40	2.3
Educational Institutions	1072	80.5	19	4.7	1091	63.0
Government	132	9.9	177	44.1	309	17.8
Hospitals	2	0.2	6	1.5	8	0.5
Religious Organizations	34	2.6	1	0.2	35	2.0
Total	1330	100.0	402	100.0	1732	100.0

Division by labor market sector and gender shows that 48.1% of workers in the deaf sector are females, whereas only 23.8% of those in the hearing sector are females (see Table 39). Looking at the situation from another angle, of the 737 women in the entire group of respondents, 637 (86.4%) are working in the deaf sector.

Of the 737 women respondents, 57.6% are teachers and another 11.8% work in human services. These data appear to support the contention that hearing-impaired women face double barriers that tend to push them into a limited selection of so-called women's jobs, jobs in such fields as teaching, social services, and nursing (Barnartt, 1982; Wax & Danek, 1982).

Oddly enough, even entry into social service positions and nursing has, until recent years, been severely limited for hearing-impaired persons. Social work has opened mainly due to the development of a degree program in social work at Gallaudet College and NTID and graduate programs (with support services) at the University of Maryland at Baltimore, New York University, and Michigan State University. These three universities specifically list their graduate programs in *College and Career Programs for Deaf Students* (Rawlings, Karchmer, & DeCaro, 1983). Other colleges and universities that accept hearing-impaired students merely say that all their courses are open to these students.

In order to discern the respondents' job satisfaction, the survey asked respondents to rate their working conditions along a continuum ranging from *like very much* to *does not apply*. Table 40 contains the responses and breaks them down according to male and female respondents. An index of job satisfaction can be calculated from these data.

Table 39
Distribution of Workers by Gender and Labor Market Sector

	Labor Market Sector					
	Deaf Sector		Hearing Sector		Total	
Gender	Number	Percent	Number	Percent	Number	Percent
Male	691	51.9	307	76.2	998	57.5
Female	641	48.1	96	23.8	737	42.5
Total	1332	100.0	403	100.0	1735	100.0

Table 40
Respondents' Ratings of Job Satisfaction
(In %)

		Working Conditions				
Respondents' Reactions	Promotion	Kind of Work	Supervision	Peers	Subordinates	Salary
Males	$n=962$	$n=989$	$n=974$	$n=970$	$n=949$	$n=975$
Like very much	41.2	76.5	57.5	71.7	52.4	42.9
Like a little	17.7	16.8	25.5	20.2	11.8	34.9
Dislike a little	5.1	5.0	6.6	2.8	1.9	12.8
Dislike very much	5.1	1.2	3.6	1.0	1.3	7.6
Does not apply	30.9	0.5	6.8	5.2	32.6	1.8
Index of job satisfaction	0.85	1.62	1.27	1.58	1.12	0.93
Females	$n=703$	$n=725$	$n=729$	$n=726$	$n=706$	$n=727$
Like very much	36.0	84.4	67.5	77.3	49.0	41.2
Like a little	14.1	10.5	19.9	17.5	11.9	33.8
Dislike a little	5.1	3.4	6.7	1.8	1.3	14.4
Dislike very much	5.0	1.4	3.2	—	0.3	10.0
Does not apply	39.8	0.3	2.7	3.4	37.5	0.6
Index of job satisfaction	0.71	1.73	1.42	1.70	1.08	0.82

The indexes of job satisfaction are weighted averages of the attitudes shown. Calculation of such an index is shown in Appendix F. A score near +1 shows a moderate liking for that particular aspect of the job; a +2 shows very high job satisfaction. Indexes lower than +1 show little satisfaction and negative indexes indicate dissatisfaction.

The scores in Table 40 show that female respondents were rather highly pleased with the human interaction (i.e., the interaction with supervisors and peers) at their jobs. The male respondents were more satisfied with promotion and salary than were the female respondents. On the overall index of job satisfaction (the sum of all indices divided by 6), women ranked a little higher than men (1.24 as compared with 1.23).

Women's tepid liking for their salaries is understandable since their median salary was $18,657 (compared to $24,503 for men). The top salary classification of $50,000 and over contained 1 woman and 27 men. This substantial difference in salaries arises from the fact that 86.4% of the female respondents work in the deaf sector. Salaries in the deaf sector average about $6,000 less than those in the hearing sector (see Table 45). Also, it is important to remember that a majority (69.4%) of the female respondents were employed in teaching or other human services, which are notoriously low-paying occupations.

The salary situation for deaf women is not unique to this study. Barnartt and Christiansen (1984), in their analysis of personal income from four studies (in 1934, 1956, 1971, and 1977), found women to be at a definite disadvantage with respect to salary. In each of the four studies, the majority of deaf women were at the lowest level of personal income. Their median incomes were also substantially less than those of deaf men in 1971 (61%) and 1977 (57%).

It has already been established that most of the jobs in the deaf sector are in the fields of education and human services and that those in the hearing sector are in government and private business. Table 41 lists the specific job categories in which respondents were employed and the percentages of respondents working in each sector. The following list contains those categories in which 75% or more of the jobs were found in one or the other sector.

Deaf Sector Jobs
Teachers, postsecondary
Teachers, except postsecondary
Counselors, education and vocational
Social and recreational workers
Religious workers
Writers, artists, entertainers, and athletes
Executive, administrative, and managerial workers

Hearing Sector Jobs
Architects
Engineers, surveyors, and mapping scientists
Mathematical and computer scientists
Health assessment and treating workers
Lawyers and judges
Health technologists and technicians
Other technicians

Two job categories in the deaf sector require some explanation. The executive, administrative, and managerial occupations include certain occupational groups that do not conform to the Census Bureau code because of their nature within the deaf community. For example, a school principal in a residential school for deaf children most likely

Table 41
Occupational Categories by Labor Market Sector
(In %)

	Labor Market Sector		
Occupational Categories	Deaf Sector	Hearing Sector	Number of Respondents
Executive, administrative, and managerial occupations	75.0	25.0	188
Management-related occupations	57.6	42.4	177
Architects	14.3	85.7	7
Engineers, Surveyors, Mapping Scientists	—	100.0	29
Mathematical and Computer Scientists	4.1	95.9	73
Natural Scientists	—	100.0	27
Health diagnosing occupations	36.4	63.6	11
Health assessment and treating occupations	—	100.0	4
Teachers, postsecondary	100.0	—	97
Teachers, except postsecondary	99.4	0.6	677
Counselors, educational and vocational	99.2	0.8	131
Librarians, Archivists, Curators	63.9	36.1	36
Social Scientists	66.7	33.3	24
Religious Workers	100.0	—	31
Social and Recreational Workers	94.3	5.7	35
Lawyers and Judges	25.0	75.0	8
Writers, Artists, Entertainers, Athletes	85.7	14.3	70
Health Technologists and Technicians	—	100.0	28
Engineering-related Technologists and Technicians	4.8	95.2	21
Science Technicians	—	100.0	1
Other Technicians[a]	15.0	85.0	60
Total			1735

[a]This category includes 49 computer programmers and 11 technicians n.e.c.

would be classified as a supervising teacher, although that classification would understate the principal's responsibilities. A superintendent in the public school system generally superintends an entire school system for a city or a section of a city; in a residential school, the position is the top managerial one in a single school, but it involves housing and dining facilities not generally the responsibility of a city school superintendent.

A number of administrators of programs involving deaf clients were accorded executive status because the administrators have unique knowledge of, and connections to, the deaf community. This tends to enlarge the responsibilities of the position. Otherwise the position might be classified as merely supervisory.

Another anomaly in the management and management-related categories is directors and coordinators of programs in institutions not existing primarily to serve deaf people (e.g., community colleges). Numerous community colleges have programs for hearing-impaired people headed by hearing-impaired supervisors/coordinators. In all, 126 of the 145 deaf sector executive positions and 86 of the 90 deaf sector management-related positions fall into these two categories.

In a similar way, the category "writers, artists, entertainers, and athletes" does not appear, on the surface, to be one in which deafness is involved. In this survey, however, there were 21 actors and directors whose deafness originally brought them into the profession; and 20 writers, editors, and public relations workers whose jobs, in the main, are related to deafness. In a related way, one of the respondents, a librarian, took a position in a city library and expanded the position into a nationwide program of deaf awareness and service.

One of the respondents who teaches hearing children gave the following reasons for why she was able to work with 30 preschool hearing children:

1. Speechreading and speech skills are very helpful.
2. The Montessori classroom teacher deals with children on a one-to-one basis, making communication easier.
3. The children are mixed ages 3–6 and stay with me 3 years, which gives them plenty of time to learn to speak slowly, facing me. If I don't understand them

even after repeats, I ask them to "show me" or another child interprets for me.
4. Each year 10 students graduate and *only 10 new ones come in.*
5. They love to use signs. Some read and use them actively. It's great for them to learn about deafness. [Respondent was severely hearing impaired before age 1, lost more hearing later, now is profoundly deaf]

Another teacher of hearing children said,

Realistically, I do enjoy teaching but I do not enjoy the job I have at present (teaching hearing third graders since 1961) because of the communication problem, so physically exhausting. . . . How nice it would be to use sign language and understand everything! [Respondent became profoundly impaired between ages 12 and 18.]

It would seem logical to assume that the less severe a person's hearing impairment is, the better able and more likely that person would be to work in the hearing sector. This assumption is not borne out by the data analyzed in Table 42. The proportions of respondents at the three levels of impairment are very similar for both sectors. However, the small differences indicate that the proportion of the less than severely impaired is a bit larger in the deaf sector than in the hearing

Table 42
Extent of Hearing Impairment by Labor Market Sector

	Labor Market Sector					
	Deaf Sector		Hearing Sector		Total	
Extent of Impairment	Number	Percent	Number	Percent	Number	Percent
Less than severe	279	21.0	65	16.2	344	19.9
Severe	246	18.5	72	17.9	318	18.4
Profound	805	60.5	265	65.9	1070	61.7
Total	1330	100.0	402	100.0	1732[a]	100.0

[a] Three respondents did not provide this information.

sector, and the proportion of profoundly impaired respondents is larger in the hearing sector than in the deaf sector.

One would think that those respondents who had acquired verbal skills before they lost their hearing would have more easily found employment in the hearing sector. The very similar proportions at each period of hearing impairment show no special sector location attributable to age of impairment. The only noticeable difference is that impairment before age 3 came to a larger proportion of respondents employed in the hearing sector (76.2%) than to those in the deaf sector (68.4%).

The means of communication used by the respondents are obviously adapted to the working situation (see Table 43). In the deaf sector, where sign language is widely used, more than half of the respondents use manual communication; in the hearing sector, where co-workers most likely are not fluent in sign language, more than half of the respondents use speech and more than 10% write.

Some tendency is apparent in Table 44 for respondents who had been in special education during high school to go into work with deaf pupils. Knowledge of the job market in the deaf sector is an obvious

Table 43
Respondents' Use of Expressive and Receptive Means of Communication in Different Labor Market Sectors

Means of Communication with Co-workers	Deaf Sector Number	Deaf Sector Percent	Hearing Sector Number	Hearing Sector Percent	Total Number	Total Percent
Expressive						
Writing	111	9.0	89	23.9	200	12.5
Talking	420	34.0	241	64.8	661	41.2
Manual means	703	57.0	42	11.3	745	46.3
Total	1234	100.0	372	100.0	1606	100.0
Receptive						
Writing	118	9.5	92	25.0	210	13.1
Talking (speechreading)	359	28.9	232	63.0	591	36.7
Manual means	764	61.6	44	12.0	808	50.2
Total	1241	100.0	368	100.0	1609	100.0

Table 44
Type of High School Respondents Graduated from and Their Labor Market Sector

	Labor Market Sector					
Type of	Deaf Sector		Hearing Sector		Total	
High School Program	Number	Percent	Number	Percent	Number	Percent
No high school diploma	9	0.7	1	0.2	10	0.6
Program for deaf pupils	795	60.1	201	50.4	996	57.9
School with no special program	510	39.0	194	48.6	709	41.2
Other[a]	3	0.2	3	0.8	6	0.3
Total	1322	100.0	399	100.0	1721	100.0

[a]This category includes correspondence school (3), high school equivalency exam (2), and tutors (1).

explanation of the choice. This situation is confirmed by Coye's research on job finding (see chap. 4). Those working in the hearing sector came in almost equal numbers from high schools with and without special programs for hearing-impaired students.

These data, of course, do not reflect respondents' attendance at elementary schools or even, in some cases, the early years at high school. Some who were deafened during later youth probably were in schools with no special program for hearing-impaired students until their hearing loss brought them into a special program. Others may have spent their elementary years in a school for hearing-impaired children but then moved into a high school with no program for hearing-impaired students.

Considering the data analyzed thus far, there appears to be little significant difference in the characteristics of the respondents in the deaf and hearing sectors, except for the gender pattern previously discussed. The records of employment in both of the sectors will be considered next.

An obvious measure of rewards from employment is salary. Comparative salaries in the two sectors are shown in Table 45. The hearing sector clearly pays better than the deaf sector. Median salaries were $20,814 per year in the deaf sector and $26,408 in the hearing sector. Median salary for the entire group was $21,957, which compares well

Table 45
Current Salaries in Different Labor Market Sectors

Salary	Deaf Sector Number	Deaf Sector Percent	Hearing Sector Number	Hearing Sector Percent	Total Number	Total Percent
Less than $10,000	42	3.2	4	1.0	46	2.7
$10,000–19,999	572	43.3	102	25.8	674	39.4
$20,000–29,999	546	41.5	142	35.8	688	40.3
$30,000–39,999	121	9.2	99	25.1	218	12.7
$40,000–49,999	30	2.3	27	6.8	57	3.3
$50,000 and over	6	0.5	22	5.5	28	1.6
Total	1317	100.0	394	100.0	1711	100.0

with the national median money income ($23,663) for professional or management workers in 1982 (Welniak & Henson, 1984).

Promotions were more frequent in the hearing sector than in the deaf sector (see Table 46). At each frequency of promotion, the proportions for the hearing sector respondents were higher. The differences in the organizational structures of business organizations and government agencies from those of schools and small service organizations is a major reason for the more frequent promotions in the hearing sector.

Less than one third of the respondents in the deaf sector had subordinates. A somewhat larger proportion of the respondents in the

Table 46
Number of Promotions by Labor Market Sector

Number of Promotions	Deaf Sector Number	Deaf Sector Percent	Hearing Sector Number	Hearing Sector Percent	Total Number	Total Percent
None	689	51.8	81	20.2	770	44.4
One	215	16.1	71	17.6	286	16.5
Two	104	7.8	63	15.6	167	9.6
Three	52	3.9	54	13.4	106	6.1
Four	30	2.3	44	10.9	74	4.3
Five or more	7	0.5	25	6.2	32	1.8
No response	235	17.6	65	16.1	300	17.3
Total	1332	100.0	403	100.0	1735	100.0

hearing sector had supervisory responsibilities. As in other analyses, the many teachers in the deaf sector colored the data. Only a few teachers reported supervising aides.

Job satisfaction needs to be measured not only in material evidence but also in jobholders' attitudes toward their working situation. Respondents were asked to rate their likes and dislikes with respect to the conditions listed in Table 47. The data are shown in percentages, but for convenience of comparison, indexes are also shown for each aspect of the job. Calculation of indexes is shown in Appendix F. Indexes range from -2 to $+2$, negatives indicating dislike and positives showing liking for that factor.

It can be seen from the indexes that job satisfaction ratings with respect to co-workers are fairly equal between the two sectors; the three

Table 47
Job Satisfaction in Different Labor Market Sectors
(In %)

Respondent Reaction	Chances for Promotion	Nature of Work	Supervisor	Co-workers	Subord- inates	Salary
Deaf Sector	$n=1279$	$n=1315$	$n=1314$	$n=1305$	$n=1272$	$n=1379$
Like very much	36.2	81.0	62.8	75.7	51.3	37.2
Like a little	14.5	13.3	22.4	17.2	11.1	33.1
Dislike a little	5.2	4.1	6.6	2.5	1.7	13.9
Dislike very much	5.3	1.1	3.6	0.5	0.7	9.5
Does not apply	38.8	0.5	4.6	4.1	35.2	6.3
Index of job satisfaction	0.71	1.69	1.34	1.65	1.11	0.75
Hearing Sector	$n=386$	$n=399$	$n=389$	$n=391$	$n=383$	$n=393$
Like very much	48.4	75.6	58.6	67.0	49.8	51.6
Like a little	21.8	17.3	25.4	25.3	14.4	33.1
Dislike a little	4.7	5.0	6.7	1.8	1.6	9.9
Dislike very much	4.1	1.8	2.6	0.5	1.3	4.1
Does not apply	21.0	0.3	6.7	5.4	32.9	1.3
Index of job satisfaction	1.06	1.60	1.31	1.57	1.10	1.18

different classes of co-workers—supervisors, co-workers, and subordinates—are all liked quite well. Subordinates received a lower rating than supervisors and peers probably because the many for whom the category did not apply reduced the level of satisfaction. Workers in the deaf sector appear to like the nature of their work a bit better than those in the hearing sector. In the hearing sector, promotion and pay brought considerably more satisfaction than they did in the deaf sector.

An overall index of job satisfaction can be calculated by summing the indexes and dividing the result by 6. This method assumes arbitrarily that each attitude has equal weight in total job satisfaction. Thus, satisfaction in the hearing sector (1.30) is a bit higher than in the deaf sector (1.21).

Table 48
Rejection Perceived by Respondents in Different Labor Market Sectors

Respondents' Perceptions	Hiring	Promotion	Training on the Job	Work Evaluation	Communication	Salary
Deaf Sector						
Very often	53	46	21	31	64	36
Often	99	97	72	78	128	93
Sometimes	308	249	203	252	359	295
Almost never	257	235	234	327	291	271
Never	532	564	686	569	420	537
Total	1249	1191	1216	1257	1262	1232
Index of discrimination	1.11	1.01	0.77	0.95	1.31	1.04
Hearing sector						
Very often	30	21	14	13	28	14
Often	39	40	30	28	23	24
Sometimes	94	112	72	83	151	95
Almost never	69	84	91	83	77	84
Never	150	123	177	176	107	165
Total	382	380	384	383	386	382
Index of discrimination	1.28	1.35	0.99	1.01	1.45	1.05

Another measure of employment satisfaction is the extent of discrimination perceived. Job satisfaction is reduced if discrimination has been experienced, no matter how interesting the work or how friendly the co-workers. Respondents were asked if they had experienced any unfair rejection in a number of job activities (see Table 48). Their perceptions were weighted from 0 (never) to 4 (very often), and the weighted sum was divided by the unweighted sum of the respondents' replies to calculate the index. Indexes were valued at 0 (never) to 4 (very often) (i.e., 4 means a great deal of unfair rejection and 0 means none).

These indexes show very little unfair rejection in any of the aspects measured. The indexes all cluster around the "almost never" category. The indexes for the hearing sector were slightly higher than those for the deaf sector, a result to be expected given the greater unfamiliarity with deafness among employers in the hearing sector. Even so, these professionals have experienced very little unfair rejection. The largest indexes of discrimination in each sector occurred for communication.

The instant supposition from the preceding paragraph probably would be that discrimination about communication occurs only among people unfamiliar with hearing impairment. This, however, would not be entirely correct. There were, and still are, schools for hearing-impaired children where the educational philosophy strongly emphasized oral/aural communication. These schools have rarely hired deaf teachers. In some schools there is tension between teachers with hearing impairments and those with none. Some of the respondents volunteered the following remarks:

> I've seen many discriminations in the circles of education and rehabilitation of the deaf . . . to obtain a higher level of professional service you have to have excellent speech skills.

> The program I am currently with has allowed only one hearing-impaired person to advance higher than a teaching position in its fifteen-plus years of existence. That person was able to use the telephone via voice and left the program after serving only one year as a counselor.

Although there have been at least three deaf persons in this program who have received MA's in education administration and supervision during the past several years and all have applied for administrative positions, all have been rejected after token interviews and without being given reasons for being passed over. In fact, outright discouragement has been voiced at their request for promotion. We have been told that "the deaf need to be realistic and seek administrative positions in a small school district first rather than in a large district such as this." However, the majority of administrators in this program began here as teachers.

I couldn't believe it that at this school most hearing teachers do not associate with deaf teachers. . . . I would rather move to a different place where there is a deaf community.

Deaf teachers of the deaf encounter an interesting experience when working alongside hearing teachers of the deaf. It is not unusual to encounter overt hostility from hearing teachers. The first time I bumped into it I thought there was something wrong with me until I talked to friends of mine around the country (R.I., Mass., Seattle, San Francisco, Texas) who had had similar experiences. The older teachers laughed and said, "It is something you must learn to live with." These are deaf teachers talking, some have learned to handle it appropriately; others have had a career change out of teaching because they couldn't handle it.

I get the distinct feeling that the hearing teacher is not aware of the hostility emanating from him/her. It's like it is a subconscious feeling covered by smiles or pleasant chatter, or simply a physical avoidance of any contacts with the deaf teacher (at meetings, parties for staff, etc.). You do learn to live with it. One has no choice. Yet, every other teacher outside the deaf program is your good friend, because they enjoy your company and you theirs.

> The thought in my mind is: If someone were to take this skeleton out of the closet and submit it to some study to verify this "experience" as being widespread, then a course of action could be taken to help all parties with it. For example, say a hearing teacher of the deaf does not like deaf adults . . . would this not hamper them in developing their own rapport with their deaf students?
>
> Likewise . . . in teacher training programs, could not the new deaf teachers be trained in ways to cope with this experience, so that their careers would not be damaged, but rather strengthened by the experience? And the same goes for hearing teachers being trained to teach deaf children. . . . They could work at being more comfortable around deaf adults, with the thought in mind that the adults are their children grown. And this way perhaps achieve a better understanding of the deaf culture to aid in their teaching.

The preceding quotations, of course, give only one side (or is it facet?) of the situation in schools for hearing-impaired children. Those with a complaint feel the urge to mention it; those satisfied do not. A few positive statements follow:

> I work at a day school program for the deaf. There is no communication problem since all teachers and staff use sign language.
>
> When I got this present job, few co-workers could use sign language. I am the only deaf teacher in this school . . . But now, most of them can use sign language.

There were complaints about the hearing sector, too.

> Severely deaf or profoundly deaf federal workers are not allowed to obtain special government driver's licenses to drive government vehicles. This serious problem really limits my chance to go on field trips aboard boats and have some chance to acquire experience.

Some federal agencies violated Sections 501 and 504 [of the Rehabilitation Act of 1973]. Today they do not care about our needs.

My present supervisor . . . said he is real satisfied with me except for communication. I asked him during my work evaluation about how to improve communication. He advised me to "read, write, and hear like hearing workers in your office."

I attended a training program for the profession of medical technology. After 10 months of training my supervisor rejected me. She refused to give me the examination [for certification]. . . . My co-workers and teachers were all very encouraging to me at this school. [The respondent now has American and international certification.]

Yesterday I talked with my supervisor and learned the real reason why I was almost not hired. My inability to hear and speak was the reason—and the others who were offered the job turned down the offer. I was the last person, therefore I was offered the job.

This corporation has training classes but they wouldn't think of hiring an interpreter. [Remark of a respondent who had been asked to give on-the-job training to a hearing-impaired worker who had language problems].

Three therapists at different times were promoted to be assistant chief over me with less experience or knowledge than mine.

The preceding quotations are not typical. They are meant to show that discrimination does exist in both sectors. It should be remembered that about 60% of the respondents in each sector never or almost never perceived unfair rejection in any aspect. In addition, 80% of the respondents said their present jobs were their dream jobs (Table 49).

Do the relatively high indexes of perceived job satisfaction and the low indexes of perceived unfair rejection mean that the respondents are

Table 49
Present Jobs and Dream Jobs Expressed in Duncan Scale Ratings

Present Job Ratings	Dream Job Ratings						
	8–39	40–49	50–59	60–69	70–79	80–89	90–96	Total
40–49	2	6	—	4	3	4	—	19
50–59	—	1	*32*	5	5	1	—	44
60–69	16	26	16	*338*	150	58	8	612
70–79	16	19	7	164	*341*	68	5	620
80–89	3	6	4	32	30	*75*	1	151
90–96	—	—	—	1	—	2	*9*	12
Total	37	58	59	544	529	208	23	1458

complacent about their jobs and do not aspire to upward mobility? As a sort of gauge of their ambitions, respondents were asked to name their dream jobs. Table 49 compares Duncan Socioeconomic Index (Blau & Duncan, 1967) ratings of respondents' present jobs and their dream jobs. The higher the Duncan score, the more prestige or status given to the job. The findings indicate that those respondents who dream of jobs with higher status than the jobs they currently hold do have aspirations to upward mobility.

The italicized figures running diagonally across Table 49 (i.e., 6, 32, 338, 341, 75, 9) represent respondents whose dream jobs correspond with the jobs they currently hold (within the range of 10 points). Of the 1,461 respondents who expressed an opinion about a dream job, 831 (54.8%) were satisfied with their present positions and did not aspire to higher levels. Those below the line and in the classification 1–39 aspired to work levels rated lower on the Duncan scale than their present positions; this group comprised 23.6% of the total. A smaller group (312, or 21.4%) aspired to positions on a higher level than their present positions. It seems clear that most of the respondents find their socioeconomic status satisfactory.

How do the aspirations of respondents in the two sectors compare? The myth is that those who face the communication barriers of the hearing sector are braver souls, the ones who face the "real" world. The data here (Table 50) do not give conclusive support to that or to any other assumption save that hearing-impaired people are people and that they react according to numerous personality variables and social situations.

Table 50
Duncan Ratings of Dream Jobs by Labor Market Sector

	Dream Job Ratings						
Sector	8–39	40–49	50–59	60–69	70–79	80–89	90–99
Deaf Sector ($n = 1332$)	18.2	3.5	4.3	28.8	33.2	11.3	0.7
Hearing Sector ($n = 403$)	17.6	2.9	1.0	39.3	22.4	13.7	3.1

Not overlooking the caveat that the dream job question might have been variously interpreted as frivolous or merely the expression of an unsubstantiated dream rather than of a serious aspiration, the data show very little variation. In the 60–79 range of the Duncan scale, the dream job ratings are almost identical for the two sectors, except that the percentages in 60–69 and 70–79 are reversed, with the deaf sector yearning for more highly rated jobs. Only at the very top do the respondents in the hearing sector tend toward higher dream jobs. There, however, the actual numbers are small, 11 persons in the deaf sector and 12 in the hearing sector.

A very few responding to this question about a dream job seized the opportunity to be fanciful. One respondent answered, "Gathering blooms from century plants." One listed multiple dream jobs: "(1) owner-operator of a hot dog stand in the Florida Keys; (2) prolific author of best-selling novels translated into the major languages of the world; and (3) hot and dusty participant in an archeological dig in the Middle East." This respondent further stated that these choices all involved "independent thought and freedom of movement," though "my present job is all I want, in truth."

Voluntary comments indicate that dream job choices reflect desire to improve personal control over working conditions, to advance one's career, to find satisfaction with the present job, and to serve hearing-impaired persons more effectively.

Summary

Neither extent of impairment nor age of occurrence seem to have been determining factors in choice of labor market sector. At least the proportions of respondents in each sector were quite similar. Job satisfaction indexes (Table 50) for the two sectors are also fairly similar—1.30 for the hearing sector and 1.21 for the deaf sector. All indexes of satisfaction are weighted means ranging between +2 (like very much) and −2 (dislike very much). (See Appendix F.)

Salary had a good deal to do with the lower index for the deaf sector; the salary satisfaction index was 0.75 compared to 1.18 for the hearing sector. The median salary for the hearing sector was $5,593 higher than that for the deaf sector. The number of persons supervised and the frequency of promotions were also higher in the hearing sector. Perceived discrimination, although generally low, was a little more frequent in the hearing sector.

As a group, these hearing-impaired professional workers are well placed, well satisfied with their occupations, and have experienced very little unfair rejection.

Chapter Six
PREDICTORS OF SOCIOECONOMIC STATUS

John G. Schroedel

The respondents in Crammatte's 1982 study represent one of the best educated groups of hearing-impaired adults ever surveyed in the United States (Schroedel, 1982a). By attending college and completing specialized training, these respondents have gained entry into high-status professional, technical, and managerial occupations. Why have these respondents become so successful? What are the key characteristics that predict their educational and occupational attainments? What kinds of occupational mobility have they experienced? How do their socioeconomic attainments compare with those of college-educated adults who hear?

Three bodies of research literature will be reviewed to help find the answers to these and related questions. The three areas are (a) studies on the influence of parental social class (i.e., socioeconomic status) on the acquisition of education and occupational status, (b) studies related to what is known as the social psychological model of status attainment, and (c) studies on the socioeconomic achievements of deaf persons.

The author appreciates the work of Afafe El-Khiami, Chris Innes, and Randy Mowry (all of the University of Arkansas) in reviewing an earlier draft of this chapter.

SOCIOECONOMIC STATUS

Every nation has a social class system, with the rich at the top and the poor at the bottom. Within a given country, social class systems change due, in part, to the expansion of trade and industry and, in part, to political revolutions. In some nations, permanent elites have ruled the social systems, preventing individuals of the lower social classes from attaining wealth, status, and power. In other countries, governments have emphasized public education and legally mandated social reforms to create opportunities for talented individuals to acquire better jobs and increased income (especially through upward mobility).

Laws, however, cannot easily change deeply rooted social practices, even in as open a society as the United States. For this and related reasons, social scientists and others have investigated how much occupational mobility there is among different social groups in the U.S., how important parental social class is in the transmission of status from one generation to another, and how important education is in obtaining good jobs and enhanced income. The findings of these investigations are important to deaf people because they can provide guidelines for public policies and new programs.

Father's level of education and occupational status are often used as indicators of parental socioeconomic status. Both of these indicators have been found to be significantly related to the educational and occupational attainments of respondents who hear (Blau & Duncan, 1967; Duncan, Featherman, & Duncan, 1972; Hauser & Featherman, 1977). Evidence shows, however, that parental social class is less influential in the deaf population than in the hearing population. The occupational status of hearing males correlated at .40 with their fathers' occupational status and their education correlated at .45 with their fathers' education (Blau & Duncan, 1967). Corresponding correlations within the deaf population were .22 and .28, respectively (Schroedel, 1976/1977).

What conditions may explain this reduction in influence of parental socioeconomic status on the attainments of deaf persons? In a study of 30 hearing-impaired female high school students, Duprez (1971) reported that there was no correlation between occupational ratings made by the subjects and those made by their parents. Duprez interpreted this to mean that even though the subjects could not correctly define parental occupational values (probably because of communication problems at home), they were still impressed by those values. The assumption can be made from Duprez's findings that hearing parents, because of their poor communication skills, cannot clearly convey to their deaf children the values and attitudes that influence academic achievement, pursuit of further education, and formation of career aspirations. Such parental values and attitudes reflect a family's socioeconomic status. To test this assumption, it is necessary to measure the quality of parent-child communication. One way to do this is to find out from whom deaf children first learn sign language.

Several studies have compared the occupational status of deaf and hearing adults to their fathers' occupational status to determine patterns of occupational mobility across one generation. Upward occupational mobility is more prevalent among the general population than it is among the hearing-impaired population. Blau and Duncan (1967) found that half of the hearing males they studied exceeded their fathers in occupational status, while Schroedel (1976/1977), in a similar study, found that only one third of the deaf workers had done so. Becoming more educated (specifically, obtaining educational credentials), increases one's prospects for upward occupational mobility. This is evident among deaf workers. Those who had completed either high school or college were more upwardly mobile occupationally than those who did not complete either high school or college (Schroedel, 1976/1977). Crammatte, in his survey of 87 deaf persons in professional employment (1968), reported that 21% had surpassed their fathers' occupational status. Quigley, Jenne, and Phillips (1968) found that among 373 hearing-impaired persons who completed college, most had exceeded their fathers in occupation, education, and overall socioeconomic status, but not income.

At every level of education, hearing workers demonstrate more upward mobility than do hearing-impaired workers. For example, among those completing 4 years of college, 69% of hearing males were occupationally upwardly mobile compared to 54% of deaf persons; among those with 5 or more years of college, 76% of hearing males were upwardly mobile compared to 57% of deaf respondents (Blau & Duncan, 1967; Schroedel, 1976/1977). Thus, deaf adults are relatively less able than their peers who hear to convert the gains of their education into higher status occupations.

The relationship between parental socioeconomic status and respondents' educational and occupational attainments is more powerful in the general population than in the hearing-impaired population. One consequence of this may be the reduced rate of upward occupational mobility of deaf persons compared to hearing persons. Inadequate communication between hearing parents and their deaf child may be a possible explanation for these patterns. The role of communication is crucial in the transmission of values and attitudes that underlie motivations to achieve. The following discussion clarifies key factors involved in this process.

THE SOCIAL PSYCHOLOGICAL MODEL

Is it true that the individuals with more abilities and drive get ahead of those with less talent and ambition? Is it also apparent that persons with more self-confidence and stronger self-concepts are more successful academically and vocationally? How important is encouragement and social support for people to do well in school and on their jobs? How do all these factors relate to each other and which are the most influential? Questions of this sort are associated with what sociologists call the *social psychological model* in research on the acquisition of educational and occupational status. This model gave researchers a needed link to the theory behind their research.

The broader roots of this theory were established by social psychologists such as Cooley (1964) and Mead (1964). They considered that an individual's self-concept developed through social interaction with significant other individuals such as parents, teachers, and peers. Super (1957) observed that an individual's self-concept was expressed through selection of an occupation or career. Educational and occupational aspirations are a central mechanism in the social psychological process formed by this model (Otto & Haller, 1979). These aspirations are created and modified through social interaction. A high school student, for example, determines his or her potential by assessing intellectual and academic abilities. Significant others also appraise these attributes and communicate corresponding expectations that influence the student's aspirations. These aspirations express ambitions as well as motivations (Porter, 1974) and are influenced by two types of significant others: *models* who exemplify appropriate educational or occupational statuses and *definers* who communicate specific expectations (Otto & Haller, 1979).

The relationships between major elements of the social psychological model are displayed in Figure 1. The location of the variables in this figure is determined by when their primary effects occur over time in the life span of an individual. Variables on the left side of the diagram are identified as early factors. Parental social class and the individual's intelligence, for example, have important influences upon a child's development and academic achievement. The arrows in the figure identify these and other patterns more clearly. A single arrow means that the variable on the left occurs before or predicts the variable on the right. Double arrows point out that the relationship between two variables is reciprocal, one variable does not precede or predict the next.

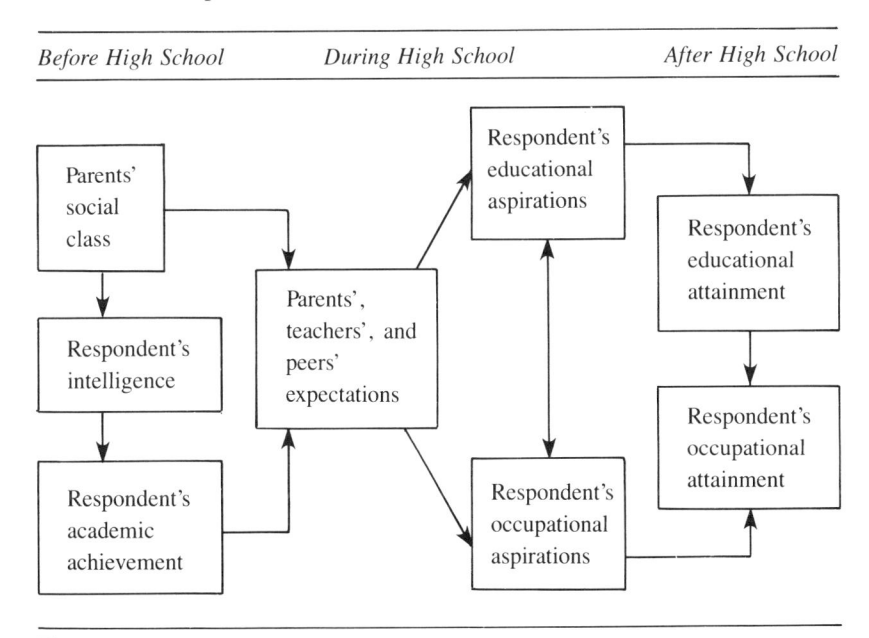

Before High School   *During High School*   *After High School*

Figure 1
Relationships Between Major Variables in the Social Psychological Model of Status Attainment

(This figure was adapted from "Schooling and Socioeconomic Attainments: High School and College Influences" by L. J. Griffin and K. L. Alexander, 1978, *American Journal of Sociology, 84,* pp. 319–347. Copyright 1978 by the University of Chicago. All rights reserved. Adapted by permission.)

Encouragement and Expectations

According to the model, a student's intelligence and academic performance directly influence the level of expectations that significant others have about that student's educational and occupational prospects. The social class level of the student's parents indirectly influences these expectations. The student, in turn, reflects upon these expectations, compares them with his or her own assessments of abilities and intelligence, then crystallizes his or her future aspirations. These aspirations then determine the ambitions underlying the pursuit of additional education and/or a job after high school.

Research studies in the general population indicate that when parents and high school personnel express expectations as encouragement for more education it has lasting and powerful effects upon youth. The amount of such encouragement is determined by such conditions as the student's intelligence, high school academic abilities, and parents' socioeconomic status (Alwin, 1974; Griffin & Alexander, 1978; Otto & Haller, 1979).

An individual's gender and race also shape the influence of educational encouragement from significant other persons, which in turn has an effect on later socioeconomic attainments. Sewell, Hauser, and Wolf (1980) found that when parents and teachers encouraged students to attend college, it directly affected the educational and occupational aspirations of these students (hearing males and females who were high school seniors in 1957). Eighteen years later, the amount of educational encouragement made by parents was evident in the educational attainments of sons, but not daughters; however, the encouragement had influenced the occupational attainments of both genders. This same study also disclosed that the educational motivation given by high school teachers influenced the 1975 educational and occupational attainments of males, but not females.

Otto and Haller (1979) found that parental encouragement was a significant predictor of the education, occupational status, and income of hearing males. The educational attainments of white males, but not black males, were significantly affected by educational encouragement from parents and peers (Porter, 1974). Fifteen years after high school, teacher expectations were found to be significantly related to the incomes of those who did not attend college, while parental expectations were significantly related to the incomes of college alumni (Griffin & Alexander, 1978). In another sample of college-educated males, the expectations of high school teachers significantly impacted respondents' income 7 years after high school (Alwin, 1974).

Type of Schooling

Other researchers have extended the social psychological model to investigate the effects of type of high school or type of college upon educational and occupational attainments. Measures of the quality of a high school may include such characteristics as the type of curriculum (vocational or academic), the number of required courses in science and mathematics, the caliber of the faculty and student body, and the level of expectations communicated by teachers and peers. Griffin and Alexander (1978) determined that characteristics of secondary schools such as those just mentioned had more significant effects on students who did not attend college than on those who did attend college. In this present study of hearing-impaired college alumni, it would be reasonable to expect that a measure of type of high school would have less impact on the group's socioeconomic achievements than would a measure of type of college. However, it is still important to include both measures to test the validity of this assumption.

Type of schooling has been an historic issue in the education of hearing-impaired youth. At the elementary and secondary level, this issue in the past focused on the relative merits of residential and nonresidential schools. In the last 10 years, the issue has centered around the advantages and disadvantages of mainstreamed education. Consequently, it is appropriate to ask whether attending a regular or special high school makes a difference in the later educational and occupational attainments of deaf adults. At the postsecondary level, the type-of-schooling issue has been expressed in terms of the benefits of special or regular colleges for hearing-impaired youth. Recent attention has also focused on the costs of special postsecondary programs such as Gallaudet College and the National Technical Institute for the Deaf (NTID) (U.S. General Accounting Office, 1985).

In the general population it is common knowledge that the 3,000 colleges and universities in the United States vary widely in the quality of education they provide. It is also well known that students are not randomly assigned to colleges. Differences in high school attended, parental socioeconomic status, as well as the student's academic abilities and motivations are significant predictors of type of college attended (Alwin, 1974; Griffin & Alexander, 1978). In addition, Alwin (1974) found that type of college made a small, but significant, difference in the socioeconomic attainments of 1,200 hearing male college alumni in Wisconsin. Considering all these factors, there is ample justification to include a measure of type of college in this present study.

Several researchers have applied elements of the social psychological model in their studies of type of schooling in the hearing-impaired population. Chubon and Black (1985) compared the career aspirations of residentially educated deaf children and regularly educated children without disabilities. They found that in the second grade both groups of children expressed similar levels in their future occupational aspirations; by the eighth grade, most of the nondisabled students desired white-collar jobs, while most of the deaf students aspired to blue-collar occupations. Joiner, Erickson, and Crittenden (1968) also reported that a majority of residentially educated hearing-impaired high school males aspired to manual occupations; however, their career aspirations were not significantly different from high school youth who could hear. Because neither Chubon and Black nor Joiner et al. controlled for important differences between the hearing-impaired and hearing students, such as parental social class, it is difficult to conclude that residential schooling is the major determinant of the career aspirations of the hearing-impaired students.

How are career aspirations formed, and what factors influence the development of these aspirations? A study by Walker (1982) of 60 teachers and 60 hearing-impaired seniors in two residential high schools sheds some light on these questions. Walker reported that teachers' expectations for their students' future occupations were the most statistically significant predictor of the students' own occupational aspirations. The students' aspirations as well as their reading abilities were, in turn, the most significant predictors of the teachers' expectations.

Walker also reported that female teachers had higher expectations for their students than did male teachers and that teachers in the academically oriented high school had higher expectations than teach-

ers in the vocationally oriented high school. This study supports at least three of the premises of the social psychological model—
1. Student abilities influence teacher expectations.
2. School characteristics influence teacher expectations.
3. Student aspirations are influenced by teacher expectations.

However, because Walker did not study important conditions such as parental social class, parental expectations, and student peer expectations, she may have overestimated the effects of teacher expectations on student occupation aspirations.

THE SOCIOECONOMIC ATTAINMENTS OF HEARING-IMPAIRED PERSONS

How do attributes of deafness relate to the educational and occupational achievements of persons who do not hear? How important is age at onset or severity of hearing loss in acquiring an education and obtaining a job? What are the influences of oral and manual communication competencies on a student's ability to complete schooling and advance in a career? How do these deafness-related variables fit into what is known about the effects of parental social class and respondents' level of education on the acquisition of socioeconomic status? Do differences due to age and sex relate to the attainments of deaf persons?

Previous research studies have identified variables associated with the educational and occupational attainments of deaf adults. Several studies on deaf persons with exceptional educational or occupational accomplishments (Crammatte, 1968; Jarvik, Salzberger, & Falek, 1963; Quigley, Jenne, & Phillips, 1968) determined that the majority of the respondents had fathers in professional or managerial occupations, were prelingually deafened, and were male. These studies also noted that a majority of deaf graduates from secondary schools with an oral communication philosophy attended regular institutions of higher education, whereas a majority of graduates from elementary and secondary schools with instruction in speech and sign language went to Gallaudet College.

A majority of Crammatte's (1968) sample attended special schools for deaf students, while a majority of those in the study by

Jarvik et al. (1963) attended regular high schools. Quigley et al. (1968) emphasized the influence of type of precollege schooling upon postsecondary education patterns. They contended that the communication philosophy of a program (oral or simultaneous) rather than the residential/nonresidential aspect of a program was a more decisive factor in these college enrollment trends. However, these authors did not fully examine how differences due to age at onset and severity of deafness, as well as student academic abilities, family background, and other important student characteristics may have influenced type of high school attended. Consequently, they may have given too much emphasis to school communication philosophy.

Schroedel (1976/1977), in analyzing a national sample of 1,100 hearing-impaired adults, reported that expressive speech skill, chronological age, and type of high school attended, in addition to fathers' education and occupational status, were significant predictors of the number of years of schooling completed. In another study, Schroedel (1982b) determined that competencies in understanding sign language, written English, and reading comprehension, as well as type of high school, severity of hearing impairment, year of college graduation, and fathers' occupational status were significant predictors of level of degree received by 713 hearing-impaired NTID graduates. Schroedel also found level of education and status of first job to be the most significant predictors of status of current occupation among these graduates.

Occupational Status

Occupational status in these studies refers to the socioeconomic status given to an occupation. This serves as an indicator of the quality of the job. After identifying which variables are significant predictors of the educational and occupational attainments of deaf persons, the next step should be to develop a framework for mapping the relationships between these variables. This framework would serve as a blueprint to design new research studies in addition to guiding the interpretation of the results of such studies in a more valid and accurate manner.

Such a framework, or model, emerged from a study by Schroedel (1976/1977) of the socioeconomic achievements of a national sample of 1,100 hearing-impaired workers. This model, displayed in Figure 2, is composed of three groups of variables: (a) those whose initial effects occur in childhood, (b) those which represent schooling factors, and (c) the educational and occupational attainments which follow.

The arrows in the figure indicate the direction of the relationship between two variables. A single arrow means that the variable on the left occurs before or predicts the variable to the right. Double arrows point out that the relationship between two variables is reciprocal, one variable does not precede or predict the next variable.

Figure 2 begins with two parental variables and two respondent variables that identify some key characteristics of the early home environment. Father's level of education and occupational status reflect parental social class. Since most respondents in Schroedel's study became deaf before 3 years of age, age at onset was classified as an early variable.

Respondents' chronological age was a significant predictor of age at onset of hearing loss; the younger respondents were more likely to have become deaf before age 3. This pattern occurred in a sample ranging in age from 16 to 65; the same pattern probably would not be found in a sample of deaf persons with a small age range.

In Figure 2, parental social class and respondents' age at onset converge upon type of early communication used by parents at home with their deaf child. As parental social class increased from low to high and age at onset occurred later rather than early, parents were more likely to use oral rather than manual methods of communication. Figure 3 also shows that the background variables are related to type of school attended by the deaf child. More specifically, those educated in special schools were more likely to have been prelingually deafened (before age 3) and come from lower-class homes than those respondents educated in regular schools.

The respondents' speech skills were affected first by the age at onset of deafness, and then by the type of parental communication. There are reciprocal effects between type of schooling and respondents' oral communication skill because it was difficult to determine which was the predecessor variable. Analyses of the data in Schroedel's study, as well as other studies reviewed, were inconclusive in respect to whether oral ability was a cause or consequence of regular or special school environments. Oral skill was found to be a significant predictor of respondents' level of education, which, in turn, was a significant predictor of occupational status.

It is important to note that Figure 2 represents a simplified map of the associations between key variables that affect respondents' level of education and consequent occupational status. The arrows indicate the most direct lines of relationships between these variables. Indirect relationships are not indicated by additional arrows because they would clutter the diagram.

Early Variables	School Variables	After School Variables

```
[Father's education]
      |
      v
[Father's occupational status]
      |
      v
[Parental communication] -> [Oral skill] -> [Respondent's education] -> [Respondent's occupational status]
      ^                       ^
      |                       |
[Respondent's age at onset of deafness] -> [Type of school]
      ^
      |
[Respondent's age]
```

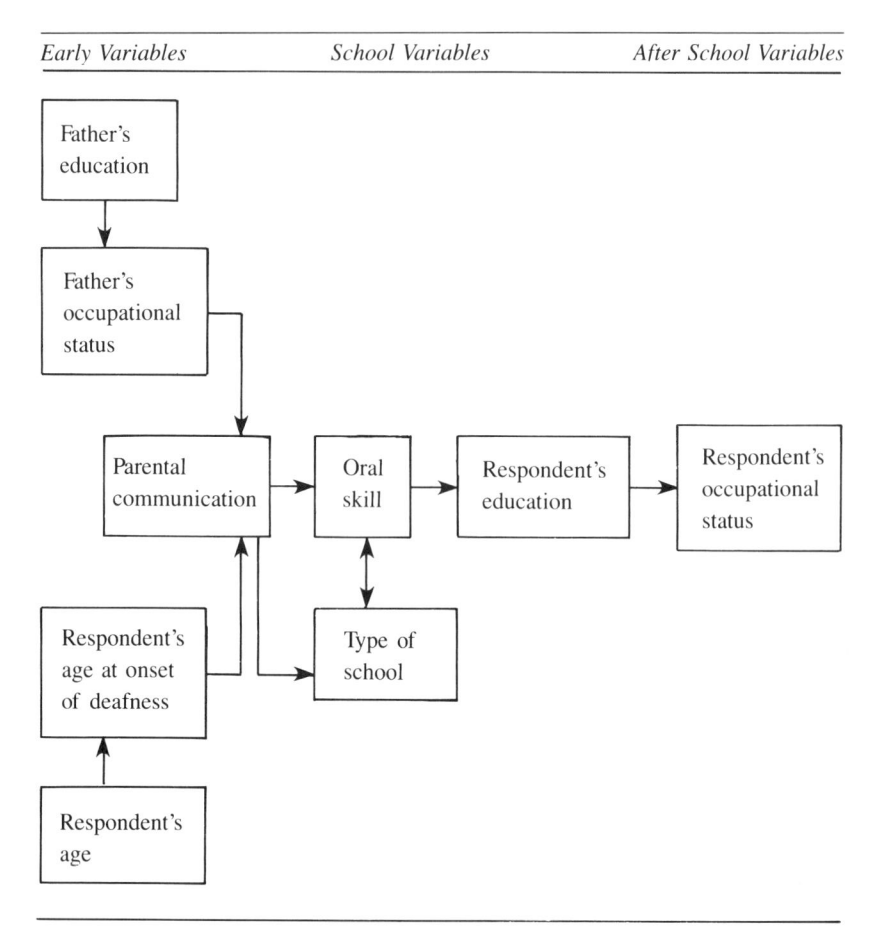

Figure 2
Relationships Between Variables Influencing the Educational and Occupational Attainments of Deaf Persons

(The data in this figure are from "Variables Related to the Attainment of Occupational Status Among Deaf Adults" by J. G. Schroedel, 1976/1977, *DAI, 38* (2), p. 1048.)

The effects of most variables in the framework are cumulative. That is, the earlier they occur (on the left side) of the diagram, the more long-term their consequences. Respondents' chronological age, for example, has an immediate effect on differences in respondents' age at onset. Chronological age also has a significant association with type of school attended, level of respondents' education, and occupational status. The best way to trace such relationships is through the arrows that link intermediate or intervening variables between two variables further apart on the diagram.

Underlying Figure 2 is the sociological process through which educational and occupational attainments result from socializing experiences at home, in school, and in the labor market. One important conclusion drawn from this model is that attributes of deafness, such as severity of hearing loss or speaking ability, predict educational accomplishments but not occupational attainments. That is, the consequences of hearing loss more directly impact schooling than they do occupational status.

One limitation must be placed on Figure 2: The model represents the results of one study. Schroedel's (1982b) research on the socioeconomic attainments of 700 deaf alumni from NTID partly replicated the model. It is possible that using a different sample of deaf adults would create a new version of the model. Therefore, it is important that additional research with other samples of deaf persons be done to test the model.

A form of this model will be tested in the current study. Variables are not available in the data set resulting from Crammatte's 1982–1983 national survey to test the social psychological model. However, key premises of this latter model are important to enlarging the context for interpreting the results of the present study.

PRELIMINARY CONCLUSIONS

The key findings from the review of the literature that are relevant to the design of the study in this chapter can be summarized as follows:
1. Research indicated that parental social class, as measured by fathers' level of education and occupational status, is an important determinant of respondents' own educational and occupa-

tional achievements. However, the effects of parental social class were found to be less powerful in the hearing-impaired population than in the general population. Inadequate communication between hearing parents and their hearing-impaired children was given as a hypothetical explanation for this pattern.
2. With the effects of parental social class reduced in the transmission of status from hearing parents to hearing-impaired child, the role of respondents' education takes on an added importance. Respondents' own level of educational attainment is in fact the single most important predictor of the status of respondents' occupation in both the general and hearing-impaired populations studied. However, at all comparable levels of education, deaf adults were less likely to be occupationally upwardly mobile than were hearing adults. It was thus concluded that deaf adults were relatively less able to convert their educational attainments into occupational attainments. To ascertain that these patterns are not limited to past samples of deaf adults studied, additional analyses will be done in this present study to (a) compare the occupational mobility patterns across one generation, (b) assess the educational and occupational attainments of different samples of college-educated adults who are deaf or hearing, and (c) compare the proportion of deaf and hearing persons in high-status professional, managerial, and technical occupations.
3. Significant others act as models and definers for the career aspirations of young adults. Their roles are variables from the social psychological research perspective; this fact may have some important implications for interpreting the results of the present study. The literature, for example, indicates that significant others have influences upon males which differ from their influences upon females. The relevancy of this finding to the current study will be discussed later.
4. The research literature points out that type of high school as well as type of college attended had significant effects upon the educational and occupational aspirations and attainments of both deaf and hearing persons. (Measures of both school variables were added to the present study.) Research also demonstrates that it is crucial to compare the characteristics of

deaf students from different types of schools before firm conclusions can be made about the possible effects that different types of schooling have on the attainments of alumni. Such analyses will also be done in this study.
5. The literature shows that variables such as severity of hearing impairment and quality of speech ability more significantly influenced the educational attainments of deaf adults than they influenced their occupational attainments. The design of the study in this chapter includes analyses to determine if these results can be replicated. In addition, age at onset of deafness, chronological age, and gender were also added to this study because prior research found them to be significant predictors of the socioeconomic attainments of hearing-impaired persons.

STUDY METHODOLOGY

Instrumentation

The assessment of occupations is a crucial element in the effectiveness of the research reported in this chapter. Lists of occupational titles such as those used by the U.S. Department of Labor (1977) or the U.S. Census Bureau (1970) do not arrange occupations into a consistent order or ranking. The Socioeconomic Index (SEI), originally developed by Duncan (1961a, 1961b) and adapted by Featherman and Hauser (1977) to the 429 occupational titles used by the U.S. Census Bureau in 1970, was selected for this study.

An SEI score represents the socioeconomic status associated with an occupation. Scale scores correlated at .57 with education and .42 with income in the general population (Duncan, 1961b) and at .45 with education and .38 with income in the deaf population (Schroedel, 1976/1977). Approximately 83% of the variance in SEI scores is due to education and income (Duncan, 1961b). Thus, the Socioeconomic Index is more than a measure of occupational prestige; it is a measure of the educational prerequisites and economic rewards of an occupation and, therefore, the social class position associated with it.

Additionally, as a metric, the SEI ranks occupations more effectively than do other scales. Many scales have been criticized for insufficiently dispersing occupations, particularly in the middle status range (Hauser & Featherman, 1977; Miller, 1970; Reissman 1959). The stratifying capacity of the SEI is demonstrated in Table 1. SEI scores range from a low of 4 to a high of 96. Manual occupations are generally rated under 39 on this scale, while clerical occupations

Table 51
The Status of Selected Occupations by Intervals of
The Duncan Socioeconomic Index

SEI Interval	Selected Occupations
4–9	Porter (4), Textile Spinner (5), Maid (6), Laborer n.e.c.[a] (8), Janitor (9)
10–19	Elevator Operator (10), Farmer (14), Cook (15), Truck Driver (15), House Painter (16), Carpenter (19)
20–29	Metal Grinder (22), Tailor (23), Bus Driver (24), Mason (27), Metal Heater (29)
30–39	Machinist (33), Plumber (34), Jeweler (36), Sales Clerk (39), Police Officer (39), Lens Grinder (39)
40–49	Library Assistant (44), Office Clerk (44), Electrician (44), Artist n.e.c. (45), Nurse (46), Clinical Laboratory Technician (48), Printer (49)
50–59	Food Store Manager (50), Bookkeeper (51), Clergy (52), Health Technician (52), Public Inspector (56), Railroad Conductor (58)
60–69	Librarian (60), Actor (60), Administrator n.e.c. (62), Elementary or Secondary Teacher n.e.c. (62), Engineering Technician (62), Technician n.e.c. (62), Social Worker (64), Computer Programmer (65), Counselor (65), Research Worker n.e.c. (65), Public Official (67), Recreational Worker (67), Draftsman (67)
70–79	Secondary Teacher (70), Designer (70), Elementary Teacher (71), Preschool Teacher (72), Office Manager (73), Archivist (75), Accountant (77), School Administrator (77), Chemist (79)
80–89	Bank Officer (80), Mathematician (80), Psychologist (81), Editor (82), Public Relations Officer (82), Civil Engineer (84), College Professor (84), Architect (85), Industrial Engineer (86)
90–96	Lawyer (92), Physician (92), Dentist (96)

Note. The data in this table are from *The Process of Stratification: Trends and Analyses* by R. M. Hauser and D. L. Featherman, 1977, New York: Academic Press. Adapted by permission. The SEI scores have been rounded to the nearest whole number.

[a]n.e.c. = not elsewhere classified.

usually are scored between 30 and 60. Professional, technical, and managerial positions generally have SEI scores above 60.

The Socioeconomic Index has been widely used by other researchers; this allows for comparisons between hearing-impaired and hearing samples. These studies, to be discussed later in this chapter, have generated comparable assessments of the occupational status of different groups at different points in time, thanks to the high stability over time of SEI scores (Duncan, 1961b; Hauser & Featherman, 1977).

Statistical Analyses

Since a primary objective of this research is to replicate the model in Figure 1, there is a need to determine which measures of the sociodemographic characteristics and deafness-related attributes of respondents are statistically significant predictors of their educational and occupational attainments. An advanced computerized procedure known as multiple regression analysis was selected for this purpose. This statistical procedure acts as a screening device that eliminates superfluous predictor variables. The effectiveness of this procedure, however, is reduced by several limitations in the present data.

The respondents in this study came from Crammatte's 1982 survey. They were employed in professional, technical, or managerial occupations that are scored on the upper half of the Socioeconomic Index (see Table 51). In addition, a majority of respondents had graduate degrees. These conditions result in a truncation in the educational and occupational measures for these respondents, especially when compared to the larger variety of measures obtainable in a broader sample of respondents. As a result, these data do not meet the ideal theoretical criterion of a multivariate normal distribution that should underlie linear regression analysis. The reduced variability of these measures limits their probability to correlate with other variables. In this study, respondents' education correlated at .14 with respondents' occupational status. In other samples of deaf workers, respondents' education correlated between .46 and .58 with respondents' occupational status (Schroedel, 1976/1977, 1982b). Respondents' education in the general population correlated at .60 with respondents' occupational status (Blau & Duncan, 1967). Consequently, as shown in the listing of simple correlations between all study variables (Table 6–A at the end of this chapter), there is a lack of high correlations between most of these variables and respondents' educational or occupational attainments. Nevertheless, the variables chosen significantly explain some of the variance in these attainments, making linear regression "a practical first approximation of a complicated relationship" (Hays, 1973).

RESULTS

Educational Attainments

Nine independent variables (numbered 1 through 8 and 10 in Table 6–A) were entered into the multiple regression analysis, the results of which are summarized in Table 6–B. Five of these variables emerged as statistically significant predictors of respondents' educational attainment as measured by number of degree-related years of college completed. As expected, three deafness-related variables—age at onset, severity of hearing loss, and speech skill—were among these leading predictors. Type of college (where respondent attended for a bachelor's degree) as well as respondents' chronological age also were significant predictors of educational attainment.

In this respect, the regression analysis achieved its primary mission of identifying significant predictor variables. Some variables were found not to be statistically significant predictors. One of these variables was *from whom first learned sign language*; better measurement of this variable may enhance its sensitivity in future analyses. Type of high school also was statistically insignificant as a predictor variable, primarily because the deafness-related variables were treated first in this analysis. Additionally, as indicated earlier in the literature review, type of high school was not expected to become a significant variable when type of college was included in the analysis. Assessments also determined that severity of hearing impairment was a falsely significant predictor of respondents' educational attainment. That is, it lacked practical significance in explaining the variance in respondents' education levels, so it was deleted from subsequent analyses.

Age at onset. The age at onset of hearing impairment has an explicit bearing on respondents' level of education (see Table 52). While 35% of those prelingually deafened (before age 3) terminated their higher education with the bachelor's degree, less than 22% of

Table 52
Distribution of Respondents' Level of Education
By Age at Onset of Hearing Loss
(In %)

Age at Onset of Hearing Loss	Number of Respondents	High School or Less	Some College	Bachelor's Degree	Master's Degree	Doctorate
Less than 1 year	950	3.1	5.6	35.3	51.8	4.2
1–2 years	253	2.4	4.7	34.8	56.5	1.6
3–5 years	204	3.4	3.9	26.0	59.8	6.9
6–11 years	171	2.3	3.5	22.8	62.6	8.8
12–18 years	67	1.5	1.5	14.9	67.2	14.9
19 years and older	67	0.0	1.5	13.4	71.7	13.4

those postlingually deafened did so. Among the six groups of respondents classified by age at onset in Table 52, educational attainment increases as does age at onset. Overall, the respondents are very well educated: 31% have a bachelor's degree, 56% have a master's, and 5% have a doctorate.

Speech skill. Speech ability is clearly associated with respondents' education level (see Table 53). About 50% of the respondents who self-rated their speech as less than good had earned a post-baccalaureate degree; nearly 70% of those with self-rated good speech had earned a post-baccalaureate degree.

The relationship between speech ability and education needs to be viewed in a broader context. Age at onset, for example, has an

Table 53
Distribution of Respondents' Level of Education by Speech Ability
(In %)

Level of Education	None n=107	Poor n=214	Fair n=488	Good n=874
High School or less	.9	4.7	3.7	2.2
Some College	9.3	6.5	6.4	2.7
Bachelor's Degree	37.4	33.2	37.1	26.3
Master's Degree	51.5	52.8	49.5	61.4
Doctorate	.9	2.8	3.3	7.4

Table 54
Distribution of Speech Ability by Age at Onset of Hearing Loss
(In %)

Age at Onset of Hearing Loss	Number of Respondents	Speech Ability			
		None	Poor	Fair	Good
Less than 1 year	915	8.7	17.6	33.9	39.8
1–2 years	246	4.5	10.2	35.4	49.9
3–5 years	200	6.5	8.5	17.5	67.5
6–11 years	169	1.2	3.6	23.7	71.5
12–18 years	67	0.0	0.0	11.9	88.1
19 years and older	66	0.0	0.0	7.6	92.4

important association with speech competencies. Specifically, self-rated speech skills were better among respondents whose hearing impairment was postlingual as opposed to prelingual (see Table 54). Forty percent of the respondents born deaf had good speech compared to 92% of those who lost their hearing after age 18. None of the respondents deafened after age 12 rated their speech less than fair, while increasing percentages of those in each earlier onset group did.

Severity of hearing loss. The significant correlation of severity of hearing impairment and speech competency is demonstrated by the data in Table 55. Eighty percent of the respondents with less than severe hearing loss rated their speech as good, compared to 45% of the respondents with more severe impairments. The overall pattern revealed in the table is that as severity of hearing loss increases, speech ability ratings decrease.

Table 55
Distribution of Respondents' Speech Skill by Severity of Hearing Loss
(In %)

Severity of Hearing Loss	Number of Respondents	Speech Skill			
		None	Poor	Fair	Good
Less than Severe	340	1.0	1.0	18.0	80.0
Severe	306	6.5	13.7	35.6	44.2
Profound	1035	7.9	16.0	31.0	45.1

Table 56
Distribution of Respondents' Level of Education by Type of College
(In %)

	Type of College	
Level of Education	Special College n=1114	Regular College n=488
High School or Less	.2	.4
Some College	.3	.8
Bachelor's Degree	36.2	26.8
Master's Degree	59.8	61.3
Doctorate	3.5	10.7

Type of college attended. The type of college that respondents attended or from which they obtained a bachelor's degree is a significant predictor of overall educational attainment. More specifically, those who attended a regular college were more likely than those who attended a special college to complete an advanced degree, especially the doctorate (see Table 56). This association between type of undergraduate college and educational accomplishment is influenced by two variables, age at onset and severity of impairment.

According to the data reported in Table 57, two thirds of the respondents educated in a special college and half of those educated in a regular undergraduate college had a profound hearing impairment. Since students with severe or profound hearing loss frequently need special support services to complete their undergraduate education, it is not surprising that 69% of all the respondents attended a special rather than a regular college.

Table 57
Distribution of Severity of Hearing Loss by Type of College
(In %)

	Type of College		
Severity of Hearing Loss	Special n=1111	Regular n=489	All Respondents N=1600
Less than Severe	14.9	33.5	20.6
Severe	19.0	16.8	18.3
Profound	66.1	49.7	61.1

Table 58
Distribution of Speech Ability by Type of College
(In %)

Speech Ability	Type of College	
	Special n = 1071	Regular n = 482
None	9.0	.4
Poor	16.7	2.3
Fair	31.3	20.7
Good	43.0	76.6

Given what is already known about severity of hearing loss and speech competency (see Table 55), it is reasonable to assume that a majority of the respondents who attended regular colleges would be better speakers than those who attended special colleges. This is confirmed in Table 58: 77% of those who attended regular colleges and 43% of those who attended special colleges had good speech. These differences in speaking abilities as well as severity of hearing impairment need to be kept in mind when comparing the educational attainments of respondents from the two types of undergraduate colleges.

Chronological age. Since respondents' chronological age was a significant predictor of their educational attainment, the relationship between these two variables was examined more closely (see Table 59). The majority of the under 25 group had obtained bachelor's degrees, while the master's had been completed by most of those over 25 years of age. Few respondents younger than age 34 had completed the

Table 59
Distribution of Respondents' Level of Education by Age Cohorts
(In %)

Level of Education	Age Cohorts						
	Under 25 n=35	25–34 n=562	35–44 n=609	45–54 n=304	55–64 n=194	Over 64 n=24	All Respondents N=1728
High School or less	0.0	.9	1.8	4.9	7.2	12.5	2.8
Some College	14.3	6.0	3.4	3.0	5.2	4.2	4.6
Bachelor's Degree	54.3	34.6	29.1	28.9	29.9	16.7	31.2
Master's Degree	31.4	56.9	59.0	55.3	50.0	58.3	56.1
Doctorate	0.0	1.6	6.7	7.9	7.7	8.3	5.3

Table 60
Distribution of Age at Onset of Hearing Loss by Age Cohorts
(In %)

Age at Onset of Hearing Loss	Under 25 n=35	25–34 n=556	35–44 n=597	45–54 n=302	55–64 n=194	Over 64 n=23
Less than 1 year	65.7	66.4	57.6	43.8	37.6	30.5
1–2 years	17.1	14.0	16.1	14.9	13.4	4.3
3–5 years	5.7	9.7	11.9	13.2	15.5	21.8
6–11 years	8.6	4.3	8.7	15.2	21.6	17.4
12–18 years	2.9	4.0	2.2	5.3	6.2	13.0
19 years and older	0.0	1.6	3.5	7.6	5.7	13.0

doctorate. The overall pattern evident in this table is that those between the ages of 35 and 54 are the best educated among the six age groups represented. It can be expected that, given time, larger percentages of those now under 35 years of age will be completing advanced degrees.

The relationship between the respondents' ages and their educational attainments needs to be analyzed in a larger setting, as both age at onset and severity of hearing impairment are also associated with chronological age. As shown in Table 60, younger respondents were more likely to be prelingually deafened than were older respondents (83% of those under 25 years of age compared to 51% of those over 54). It follows, then, that as the age of the respondents increases, so does the percentage of those who became postlingually deafened.

There is a statistically significant correlation between chronological age and severity of hearing impairment. Table 61 shows the relationship between these two variables. The main result seen in this table is that respondents under 35 years of age were somewhat less severely hearing impaired than were older respondents. The older respondents tended to be severely or profoundly hearing impaired.

Analysis. A number of significant predictors of respondents' level of education have been identified and discussed. These predictor variables include age at onset of hearing impairment, severity of hearing impairment, chronological age, speech ability, and type of college attended. In addition, several important relationships between certain key predictors (e.g., chronological age and age at onset; chronological age and severity of hearing impairment) were also found.

Table 61
Distribution of Severity of Hearing Loss by Age Cohorts
(In %)

	\multicolumn{7}{c}{Age Cohorts}
Severity of Hearing Loss	Under 25 n=35	25–34 n=562	35–44 n=607	45–54 n=304	55–64 n=194	Over 64 n=24	All Respondents N=1726
Less than Severe	22.9	24.6	17.5	18.8	16.0	8.3	19.8
Severe	17.1	19.9	20.8	16.1	8.8	33.3	18.4
Profound	60.0	55.5	61.7	65.1	75.2	58.4	61.8

These and other relationships should be considered when interpreting the patterns found among these significant predictor variables and respondents' education. These patterns will be discussed more completely at the end of this chapter.

Occupational Attainments

Ten variables (numbered 1 to 10 in Table 6–A) were entered into a regression analysis to determine which were statistically significant predictors of respondents' occupational status. The results appear in Table 6–C. Three of the 10 variables—respondents' education, gender, and fathers' occupational status—emerged as statistically significant predictors of occupational attainment.

Level of education. Table 62 demonstrates how respondents' educational level relates to their occupational status. The major finding in this table is that median occupational status scores increased as respondents' level of education increased. These medians closely resemble the distribution of respondents across the SEI range for each of the five educational categories in the table.

A majority of the respondents who neither attended college nor completed a bachelor's degree had jobs in the 60–69 SEI bracket. A majority of those who had earned bachelor's degrees were also in this bracket. The greatest percentage of master's degree recipients were in the 70–79 SEI bracket. That the median SEI scores for the bachelor's and master's degree groups are similar is not surprising when one considers that society values scientific and technological (not necessarily technical) occupations more than teaching or human services.

Table 62
Distribution of Respondents' Occupational Status
By Level of Education
(In %)

Level of Education	Number of Respondents	Occupational Status 40–59[a]	60–69	70–79	80–96[b]	Median Score
High School or Less	48	10.4	64.6	14.6	10.4	64.6
Some College	81	11.1	60.5	23.5	4.9	64.1
Bachelor's Degree	537	6.0	48.8	35.7	9.5	66.7
Master's Degree	970	3.5	39.0	48.3	9.2	68.0
Doctorate	91	1.0	18.7	35.2	45.1	75.0
All Respondents	1727	4.7	42.7	41.6	11.0	67.7

[a] The 40–49 SEI interval (with 26 respondents) was combined with the 50–59 interval (with 53 respondents).
[b] The 80–89 interval ($n=175$) was also combined with the 90–96 interval ($n=15$).

An engineer with a BS degree obtains an SEI score of 84, a teacher with an MA degree earns a 72, and a counselor with an MA obtains an SEI score of 65.

The median occupational status score for respondents with doctorates was the highest among all respondents. Forty-five percent of doctorates were in the highest rated (80–96) occupations. The 80–89 SEI interval represents the upper limit for most respondents because only 8% of all respondents were actually in occupations rated between 90–96. In other words, less than 1% of all survey respondents had occupations rated above 89 on the SEI scale. The reasons for this underrepresentation of hearing-impaired adults in the highest rated occupations will be discussed later in this chapter.

Two other patterns are noteworthy in Table 62. One is that 84% of all respondents were clustered in the 60–79 ranges of the SEI. The other is the variability of SEI ranges: 18.7% of the respondents with doctorates were in occupations rated between 60 and 69, while 10.4% of those without any college education were in the highest occupational status category (80–96). Most of these latter respondents have probably advanced to their current positions through extensive on-the-job training, self-instruction, work experience, career tenure, and other non-academic forms of developing human capital.

Gender. Table 63 clarifies the relationship between respondents' gender and occupation. Most females were employed in occupations traditionally held by women. Fifty-eight percent of the female respondents were teachers, compared to 35% of the male respondents. The percentages of females also exceeded males in counseling, library science, social-recreational work, nursing, and health technologies.

Hearing-impaired female respondents were underrepresented in administrative and managerial-related positions, engineering, the natural sciences, computer technology, mathematics, and medicine, all traditionally male occupations. Males also surpassed females in most technical occupations. Apparently, it is not the occupational category, (e.g., professional or technical) that creates the gender patterns in Table 63 so much as it is the orientation of occupations—scientific/technological vs. educational/human services. This orientation evidently contributes to occupational clustering by gender among not only hearing-impaired respondents, but also in the general labor force (Bureau of the Census, 1981).

The influence of gender on selection of college majors may help explain why hearing-impaired males and females enter particular occupations. Cook and Rossett (1975) reported that deaf male and female undergraduates at Gallaudet and NTID chose majors they perceived to be appropriate for their gender. Business administration, mathematics, accounting, engineering, computer science, scientific or manufacturing technologies, printing, and photography were the dominant selections made by males. Home economics, social work, English, psychology, office or clerical practices, and medical technologies were chosen by the majority of females. At technical-vocational institutes in St. Paul, Seattle, and New Orleans, deaf students followed similar patterns—majorities of females enrolled in clerical training, while majorities of males trained in the skilled crafts (Harlow, Fisher, & Moores, 1974).

The development of educational and counseling strategies to change these occupational patterns among hearing-impaired males and females has been preceded by research studies focusing on attitudes towards social roles and occupations. Comparing hearing-impaired and hearing high school-aged females, Cook and Rossett (1975) found that the former had more traditional attitudes than their hearing peers towards marriage, child rearing, and work. At the postsecondary level, deaf males expresed significantly more conservative opinions on gender responsibilities in social roles than than did hearing males (Kolvitz & Ouellette, 1980).

Among junior high school students, hearing-impaired males and females were three times more likely than their same-aged peers who hear to stereotype occupations by gender; that is, to view jobs as exclusively either for males or for females (Kovolchuk & Egelston,

Table 63
Distribution of Respondents' Occupations by Gender
(In %)

Respondents' Occupations	Male N=998	Female N=737
Teachers, elementary and secondary	29.2	52.6
Teachers, postsecondary	5.9	5.2
Counselors	6.7	8.7
Librarians, Archivists	1.1	3.4
Social and Recreational Workers	1.2	3.1
Religious Workers	3.0	.1
Managers and Administrators	13.9	6.8
Managerial-related[a]	12.2	7.5
Engineers, Surveyors, Cartographers	2.9	0.0
Architects	.6	.1
Mathematicians, Computer Scientists	6.2	1.5
Natural Scientists	2.5	0.3
Psychologists	1.1	1.6
Doctors, Dentists	1.0	0.1
Nurses, Therapists	0.0	0.5
Lawyers, Judges	0.5	0.4
Writers, Artists, Actors	4.6	3.3
Health Technicians	1.1	2.3
Engineering Technicians[b]	2.0	0.1
Scientific Technicians	0.0	0.1
Other Technicians[c]	4.3	2.3

[a] Includes accountants, purchasing agents, auditors, buyers, inspectors.
[b] Includes graphic designers, draftsmen, engineering technicians, and surveying technicians.
[c] Includes computer programmers, legal assistants, and other technicians not elsewhere classified.

1976). While hearing-impaired females were more likely than hearing-impaired males in junior high school to have gender stereotypes about jobs (Egelston, 1974), hearing-impaired male freshmen at NTID were significantly more likely than their female classmates to apply gender stereotypes to occupations (Egelston-Dodd, 1977a). NTID students of either gender who viewed occupations by gender labels also were more likely to view occupations by hearing ability (i.e., considering occupations as more suitable for hearing than hearing-impaired workers). Actual labor market patterns contradict such stereotypes.

Taken as a whole, these studies suggest that many hearing-impaired youth of both genders possess traditional stereotypic attitudes about gender in relationship to social roles and occupational choices. Compounding these traditional attitudes is a tendency to impose perceived limitations due to deafness upon attitudes towards occupations. The perpetuation of gender stereotypes in occupational choices requires solutions.

One of the immediate goals should be to change the attitudes and behaviors of hearing-impaired youth through well-developed self-awareness and career learning courses in secondary (Cook & Rossett, 1975) as well as postsecondary programs (Egelston-Dodd, 1977a). Science education programs should be infused into all levels of the educational curriculum (Egelston-Dodd, 1977b, 1978). For hearing-impaired adults, especially women, Wax and Danek (1982) advocated the use of new counseling strategies to develop skills and attitudes to overcome traditional role barriers and sexist stereotypes to cope more effectively with both home and career activities.

These strategies can be strengthened by research on the social psychological model to better understand the factors that influence the formation of educational and occupational aspirations among deaf adolescents. Knowledge from such research could then be applied to increase the effectiveness of parents and teachers in increasing the self-awareness and occupational awareness of deaf youth.

The research literature suggests that hearing parents have a limited amount of influence on the career aspirations of their hearing-impaired children. The reasons for this include (a) the fact that residential education separates the child from home and (b) the reality that there is often inefficient communication between parents and their deaf children (Lerman & Guilfoyle, 1970).

Other research points out that parental occupational expectations are not very optimistic. Munson and Miller (1979) reported that parents believed that deafness limited job opportunities for their deaf children. Meadow (1967) found that a majority of hearing parents thought that deaf people could not succeed as well as hearing people did in employment. She also reported that hearing parents had lower occupational expectations for their deaf children than deaf parents had for their deaf children.

The deaf subculture may be a conduit for the transmission of vocational information and aspirations among hearing-impaired youth. Lerman and Guilfoyle (1970) observed that ideas about work are communicated from the adult deaf community to older deaf students, who in turn pass them on to younger deaf students. However, research is needed to confirm this observation. In addition, the dynamics that influence the career aspirations of residentially educated and nonresidentially educated hearing-impaired students need to be compared. Then the effects of type of schooling can be specified more accurately. The literature presently suggests that deaf youth in residential schools have limited exposure to a variety of occupational role models (Chubon & Black, 1985; Lerman & Guilfoyle, 1970). This may be one reason why teaching is the leading occupation for both male and female respondents in this study.

While gender was not a statistically significant predictor of respondents' educational accomplishments in this study, it still may be worthwhile to ask, Were there gender differences in educational attainments that may help explain gender differences in occupational attainments? While 63% of the female respondents and 51% of the male respondents had obtained a master's degree, 8% of these men, compared to less than 2% of the women had completed a PhD (see Table 64). The excess of males over females at the doctoral level affects occupational status more than the excess of females over males at the MA level. Most of the women with MAs have become elementary and secondary school teachers or counselors. These occupations are rated between 65 and 72 on the SEI. Most of the men with PhDs have entered higher status occupations.

Increasing the number of hearing-impaired women with earned doctorates would be a key step in removing the gender inequalities in occupational status among highly educated hearing-impaired adults

Table 64
Distribution of Respondents' Level of Education by Gender
(In %)

Level of Education	Males N = 998	Females N = 737
High School or Less	3.6	1.6
Some College	5.1	4.1
Bachelor's Degree	32.6	29.2
Master's Degree	50.7	63.5
Doctorate	8.0	1.6

such as those in this survey. Additionally, barriers in the general society need to be identified and modified to achieve this goal. Stated differently, among the 92 survey respondents with earned doctorates, 80 (or 87%) were males. This proportion is comparable to the distribution of doctorates by gender in the general population. According to the 1981 Survey of Doctoral Recipients, there were 340,900 scientists and engineers with doctorates, as well as 67,000 workers with doctorates in the humanities employed in the general labor force during 1981 (Maxfield, 1982). Among the scientists and engineers, 88% are male; among those with a doctorate in the humanities, 73% are males.

In the sample for the 1979 Survey of Doctoral Recipients, 893 of the 23,000 respondents (3.9%) reported a handicap. Of this group, 172 had an auditory impairment (B. D. Maxfield, personal communication, February 12, 1982). Despite the scientific difficulties in conducting a census of disabled people, the best current estimate (Haber & McNeil, 1983) is that between 8.5% and 17% of the U.S. population is disabled (Albrecht & Levy, 1984; Haber & McNeil, 1983; Schroedel & Jacobsen, 1978).

In essence, these statistics convey one message: Disabled Americans, including those with hearing impairments, are underrepresented among Americans with earned doctorates. Changing this situation will require a focused effort on developing a common cause centered on the disability issue. This effort might be more powerful and more beneficial than limiting the effort to gender issues.

Father's occupational status. The third significant predictor of respondents' occupational status was their fathers' occupational status. Comparisons were made between fathers' and sons' occupational status

(Table 65) and between fathers' and daughters' occupational status (Table 66).

The respondents were asked to report their mothers' and fathers' occupations when the respondents were 16 years old (see Appendix C). Because 58% of the mothers were reported as not working, only the fathers' occupation was used to determine the family's socioeconomic status. The median Socioeconomic Index score of the 732 working mothers was 44; the median score for fathers was 50. A score of 4–39 corresponds to the lower class; a score of 40–69 corresponds to the middle class; and a score of 70–96 to the upper class (Perrucci & Perrucci, 1970). While most of the respondents came from middle class homes, there was some variety in their parents' socioeconomic status.

It is useful to recall that the specific type of occupational mobility examined here is mobility over one generation. This technique compares the status of the respondent's occupation to the status of his or her father's occupation to determine whether the respondent has been

Table 65
Distribution of Males' Occupational Status
By Occupational Status of Their Fathers
(In %)

Fathers' Occupational Status	Number of Respondents	40–59[a]	60–69	70–79	80–96[b]
1–9	19	21.1	15.8	47.3	15.8
10–19	206	5.3	37.9	46.2	10.6
20–29	79	5.1	46.9	39.2	8.8
30–39	78	2.6	47.4	41.0	9.0
40–49	78	*9.0*	41.0	34.6	15.4
50–59	110	*4.5*	47.3	36.4	11.8
60–69	195	3.1	*41.0*	41.5	14.4
70–79	66	6.1	36.4	*34.8*	22.7
80–89	72	4.2	40.3	34.7	*20.8*
90–96	41	12.2	31.7	36.6	*19.5*
All	944	5.4	40.8	40.0	13.8

[a]The 40–49 SEI interval (with 26 respondents) was combined with the 50–59 interval (with 53 respondents).
[b]The 80–89 interval ($n = 175$) was also combined with the 90–96 interval ($n = 15$).

Table 66
**Distribution of Females' Occupational Status
By Occupational Status of Their Fathers
(In %)**

Fathers' Occupational Status	Number of Respondents	Females' Occupational Status			
		40–59[a]	60–69	70–79	80–96[b]
1–9	16	—	50.0	50.0	—
10–19	134	2.2	52.2	41.1	4.5
20–29	47	—	51.1	46.8	2.1
30–39	39	2.6	43.6	46.1	7.7
40–49	40	2.5	42.5	45.0	10.0
50–59	108	*1.9*	45.4	48.1	4.6
60–69	162	5.6	*37.7*	46.8	9.9
70–79	64	4.7	43.7	*39.1*	12.5
80–89	62	3.2	51.6	38.7	6.5
90–96	31	12.9	38.7	41.9	6.5
All	703	3.6	45.2	44.2	7.0

[a]The 40–49 SEI interval (with 26 respondents) was combined with the 50–59 interval (53 respondents).
[b]The 80–89 interval ($n = 175$) was also combined with the 90–96 interval ($n = 15$).

upwardly mobile, immobile, or downwardly mobile across one generation. It is also important to note that the selectiveness of this survey sample constrains in-depth discussion of mobility patterns. Since all respondents in this survey were employed in professional, technical, or managerial jobs, no respondent had an SEI score below 40. However, 40% of the males and 34% of the females had fathers with occupations below 40 on the SEI (see Tables 65 and 66). Many of the respondents from lower-class homes with fathers in manual occupations achieved high-status jobs through opportunities in higher education.

The occupational patterns of respondents with fathers ranked 40 or higher on the SEI can be discussed with more precision. In Tables 65 and 66, the italicized percentages in each of the rows of SEI scores 40 or higher indicate the proportion of respondents in that row whose occupations are similar in status to their fathers. These people are considered to be occupationally immobile. Percentages to the left of the underlined figure represent downward mobility; percentages to the right indicate upward mobility.

Tables 65 and 66 show that most males and females, respectively, with fathers in the 40–49 and 50–59 SEI intervals were occupationally upwardly mobile. A smaller number of both genders with fathers in the 60–69 interval have also experienced upward mobility. Among males and females having fathers with occupations rated 70 or higher on the SEI, a majority of both genders have encountered downward occupational movement over time.

The findings from Tables 65 and 66 can be summarized as follows:

1. The 40% of males and 34% of females with fathers who had SEI scores under 40 have experienced extensive upward mobility into professional and related occupations.
2. Most of the 40% of males and 44% of females with fathers whose SEI scores range between 40 and 69 have also experienced upward mobility.
3. A large majority of the 20% of males and 22% of females with fathers whose SEI scores were 70 or higher have, as a group, experienced downward mobility.
4. Overall, a majority of all males and females have experienced upward occupational mobility over one generation.

From these findings the conclusion can be made that fathers' occupational status has a direct influence on how much occupational mobility, be it upward, stable, or downward, respondents have encountered. Understanding these patterns sheds some light on what is known as the American social class structure. When parental social class is a key determinant of how well children have fared in education and employment as adults, this is called *social-distance mobility* (Theodorson & Theodorson, 1969). In contrast, technological and economic forces create *demand mobility*, which is the expansion of professional, managerial, and other white-collar job opportunities with a reduction in the need for manual workers (Rogoff, 1953).

The United States remains an open class system because of both types of mobility, one partially due to social class and the other partially due to changes in the economy. However, the key to socioeconomic equality for all social groups is equal access to higher education. Neither the amount of social-distance mobility nor the amount of demand mobility among hearing-impaired respondents can be specified with the current data. Clearly, respondents have experienced both types of mobility. The central point is that their high level of educational attainment has been a major reason for their overall gains in occupational status. There are reasons to believe that these gains are due more to the respondents' education than to their fathers' occupational status. The justification for this and related conclusions will be made at the end of this chapter.

A final observation can be made from Tables 65 and 66: 14% of the male respondents and 7% of the female respondents have occupations in the highest SEI category (80–96). At each interval of fathers' occupational status from 1–9 to 90–96 on both tables, larger proportions of males over females were found in the highest rated occupations. Two reasons combine to create this overall pattern—one is the underrepresentation of women with doctoral degrees; the other is the preference by more males than females for scientific and technological careers rather than education and human service careers. This preference gives a disproportionate number of men access to higher status professional jobs.

COMPARISONS TO OTHER SAMPLES

Hearing-Impaired and Hearing College Alumni

How do the current survey respondents compare to other samples of college-educated adults who are hearing impaired? How do hearing-impaired college alumni compare to hearing persons with a college education? Some answers to these questions are provided by data on the educational and occupational attainments of nine samples of hearing-impaired and hearing adults (see Table 67).

Differences in education account for most of the variation in occupational attainments among four samples of hearing-impaired college alumni. Crammatte's 1983 survey respondents had the highest mean occupational status score in part because they were the best educated among these four groups. In fact, mean Socioeconomic Index scores declined among these four samples as mean level of education declined. Eighty percent of the NTID/RIT graduates had completed postsecondary vocational or associate degree programs (Schroedel, 1982b). The college-educated subsample from the 1971 National Census of the Deaf Population included those who had attended college without graduating (Schroedel, 1976/1977). All other samples of hearing-impaired alumni in Table 67 were college graduates. The high socioeconomic attainments of the 1983 survey respondents also reflect the fact that these hearing-impaired adults represent a selective sample. The main criterion for their inclusion in the survey was that they were employed in a professional, technical, or managerial job. Fifteen percent of the hearing-impaired Gallaudet graduates surveyed in 1980 were not employed in these occupational categories; among nongraduating Gallaudet alumni, 79% of males and 70% of females were employed in clerical and manual jobs (Armstrong, 1983). Similar patterns occur in the general population.

Thirty-four percent of hearing persons who graduated from college between 1969 and 1978 with a bachelor's degree found employment in job catetories other than professional, technical, and managerial (Bureau of Labor Statistics, 1980). These conditions need to be kept in mind when comparing the samples of hearing-impaired and hearing adults in Table 67.

The most striking trend in Table 67 is that in almost every comparison between hearing-impaired and hearing college alumni at similar levels of education, those who hear surpassed the occupational attainments of those who cannot hear. The differences in mean Socioeconomic Index scores in these comparisions in Table 67 range between .1 and 10.7 points on the 92–point SEI. The average difference is 4.7 SEI points in favor of the samples of hearing adults. For example, the hearing-impaired male respondents in Sample 1 had an average SEI score significantly below that of the corresponding group of hearing males in Sample 7. Also, deaf male graduates of NTID (Sample 2) had a mean SEI score lower than the comparably educated hearing male college alumni in Samples 5, 6, and 8.

There is a paucity of comparable research studies on the socioeconomic attainments of women with a college education. This is unfortunate because increasing numbers of college-educated women have been entering the professions in recent years. The hearing-impaired females in Sample 1 had a mean SEI score a bit higher than the mean score of the hearing females in Sample 9. However, there was nearly one year's difference in mean education between the two groups primarily because 65% of the hearing-impaired females had graduate degrees compared to 12% of the hearing females.

Table 67
Educational and Occupational Status for College-Educated Adults
Who Are Hearing Impaired or Hearing: United States, 1962–1983

Sample Populations	N	Mean Education	Occupational Status Respondents' Mean	(S.D.)	Fathers' Mean
1. Deaf males, 1983	995	17.0	70.6	(8.8)	46.8
Deaf females, 1983	733	17.0	69.6	(7.2)	49.9
2. Deaf males, NTID 1979–1980	379	15.3[a]	54.8	(17.9)	
Deaf females, NTID 1979–1980	226	15.3[a]	52.6	(14.9)	51.1[b]
3. Deaf males and females, Gallaudet, 1980	1290	16.7	64.8[c]	—	—
4. Deaf males and females, Gallaudet, 1971	136	15.1	50.7	(23.2)	—
5. Hearing males, 1970	668	15.0	58.1	(20.1)	—
	2795	16.0	66.9	(17.3)	—
	802	17.0	70.7	(16.0)	—
6. Hearing males, 1972	365	15.4	61.5	(16.0)	37.7
1975			61.1	(16.3)	
7. Hearing males, 1962	3256	16.0	66.6	—	43.1
	2276	17.0	74.0	—	47.6
8. Hearing males, 1964	1198	15.1	56.5	(22.7)	—
Tech Institute Alumni	83	15.5	65.5	—	—
9. Hearing males, 1964	1369	16.2	73.3	(14.2)	46.0
Hearing females, 1964	758	16.1	67.7	(11.2)	53.7
10. Hearing males, 1970	525	16.2	62.9	(20.7)	45.8

Note. Status of respondents' and fathers' occupations was based on the Duncan Socioeconomic Index. In most samples, status of fathers' occupation was when respondent was 16 to 20 years of age. Respondents' occupational status was for current job at time of survey. Mean education under 16.0 refers to number of years of education; means 16.0 and higher are degree-related years of education.

The data in samples 2–10 come from the following sources:

2—NTID graduates between 1969–1978, 23–31 years of age in 1980 (Schroedel, 1982a);
3—Gallaudet graduates, median age = 39 in 1980 (Armstrong, 1981);
4—From 1971 National Census of the Deaf Population, 18–64 years of age (Schroedel, 1976/1977);
5—From U.S. Census 1/1000 public use sample, 25–64 years of age (Jencks et al., 1979);
6—From 1972 Panel Study of Income Dynamics, heads of households, 25–60 years of age (Trusheim & Crouse, 1980, 1981);

The differences in the dates of the samples compared in Table 67 do not affect the conclusions drawn from the data presented. As educational attainment in the population increases over time, comparisons between recent samples of deaf persons and previous samples of hearing persons would favor the former over the latter. Occupational status in the general population has increased as people have become better educated. As measured by the SEI, mean occupational status increased about three scale points for hearing males between 1962 and 1973 (Featherman & Hauser, 1975).

As discussed earlier in this chapter, the SEI is a measure of one's social class. It is a summary of the material resources at one's command as well as an indicator of the quality of life one possesses. For hearing and hearing-impaired people, a lower score on the SEI can be directly translated into reduced income, lower quality of housing, less education, and other measures of social class (Blau & Duncan, 1967; Schroedel, 1976/1977). That the cream of the nation's crop of hearing-impaired adults have not yet obtained socioeconomic parity with their similarly educated counterparts who hear should raise concerns.

Gender

In addition to comparisons based on the hearing status of respondents, Table 67 allows comparisons on the basis of gender. In Samples 1 and 2, the hearing-impaired males exceeded the hearing-impaired females in occupational attainments. In Sample 9 hearing males had a higher SEI score than did hearing females. One explanation of this is that males obtain employment in a wider range of jobs than do females. Comparisons of standard deviations (SDs) for SEI scores across relevant survey samples support this explanation. The standard deviations

---

Table 67 Notes *(continued)*

7—From 1962 Occupational Change in a Generation I survey, non-Black males from nonfarm backgrounds (Blau & Duncan, 1967; Duncan, Featherman, & Duncan, 1972);
8—From Wisconsin sample of 1957–1964 college alumni (Alwin, 1974);
9—From 1968 NORC panel survey of 1961 college graduates (Perrucci, 1978);
10—From 1970 follow-up survey of a national sample who were high school sophomores in 1955, conducted by Educational Testing Service (Griffin & Alexander, 1978).

[a]Number of years of education (see Di Lorenzo & Welsh, 1981).
[b]Combined mean SEI score for fathers of males and fathers of females.
[c]Mean SEI estimated from converting occupational category titles from 1977 Directory of Occupational Titles to 1970 U.S. Census Bureau codes then to SEI scores.

for SEI scores of hearing-impaired males and females in Sample 1 were relatively small because of the selectivity of this sample. The standard deviation for hearing-impaired females in this sample was 82% of that for hearing-impaired males. Among the NTID graduates in Sample 2, the standard deviation of hearing-impaired females was 83% that of hearing-impaired males.

Hearing females experience similar restrictions in their labor market. In Sample 9, the standard deviation for females was 79% the size of the standard deviation of males. In another study of college alumni who hear, the standard deviation for occupational status of females was 74% (Spaeth, 1977). There is evidence that college-educated females in the general population have interrupted careers because of marriage and child rearing. Many of these women tend to be employed in occupations such as teaching, where departure from and return to employment is relatively easy (Spitze & Spaeth, 1977). There are clear reasons to believe that hearing-impaired women who are college educated experience similar patterns in fulfilling their roles as workers, wives, and mothers. Future research studies can explore these circumstances more deeply, particularly in view of more recent trends in the labor market. The fact remains that limitations in the range of occupations open to women do indeed reduce the career attainments of women.

High Status Occupations

Restricted access to occupations, specifically those that are highest in socioeconomic status, partially explain why hearing-impaired adults lag in occupational achievement behind their college-educated peers who hear. More than 70% of Crammatte's 1983 survey respondents were employed in the deaf sector of the labor market (see Table 38, p. 74). Among Crammatte's 1,330 respondents, 836 (63%) were working as elementary and secondary school teachers, counselors, or social and recreational workers (see Table 41, p. 78). SEI scores for these occupations (see Table 51) are below the average SEI score of 75 for all professional and technical occupations (Hauser & Featherman, 1977).

Except for the 97 hearing-impaired respondents employed as postsecondary teachers, relatively few other respondents were clustered in the occupations with the highest SEI scores. As demonstrated in

Table 68, hearing-impaired respondents to the 1983 survey were less likely to be employed in occupations rated at the highest levels of the Socioeconomic Index.

The key statistic in Table 68 is the ratio of hearing-impaired workers per 100,000 hearing workers in selected professional jobs. Not surprisingly, these ratios were most favorable for deaf workers in the educational fields and in mathematics and computer occupations. These ratios were at intermediate levels for the next five occupations in the table—architecture, chemistry, psychology, social work, and accounting. Each of these occupations has an SEI score between 65 and 85. The proportions of hearing-impaired respondents in the highest-

Table 68
Numerical Distributions of Hearing-Impaired and
Hearing Persons in Selected Professional Occupations

Occupation (SEI scores)	Hearing Impaired	Hearing[a]	Rate per 100,000 Hearing[b]
Total Population	410,522[c]	207,000,000	203
Elementary and secondary teachers (70–72)	677	2,438,000	28
Mathematicians (80)	9	38,000	24
Computer Programmers and Analysts (65)	103	497,000	21
Postsecondary Educators (84)	95	717,000	13
Architects (85)	8	70,000	9
Chemists (79)	15	166,000	9
Psychologists (81)	12	159,000	8
Social Workers (65)	27	417,000	6
Accountants (77)	61	1,229,000	5
Dentists (96)	4	144,000	3
Engineers (84)	28	1,322,000	2
Lawyers (92)	7	635,000	1
Physicians (92)	3	481,000	1

[a] Data on numbers of persons who hear in selected professional occupations projected to 1983 obtained from Bureau of Labor Statistics (1980; passim).
[b] Ratio is defined as number of hearing-impaired persons per 100,000 hearing persons.
[c] Prevalence data represents the number of persons who became deaf by age 19 in the 1971 population. This prevocationally deaf population is the most comparable to the survey respondents—96% became deaf before age 19; 80% have Hearing Ability Scale scores similar to those in the 1971 National Census of the Deaf Population.

rated professional occupations—dentistry, engineering, law, and medicine—were at token levels.

The data in Table 68 are incomplete because the 1983 mail survey was not a national census of all severely hearing-impaired Americans in professional, technical, and managerial positions. However, considering the degree of effort invested in name list building and the 66% rate of survey response (see Appendix A), such a census probably would not dramatically change the overall order of results found in the table.

Education and Mobility

Mean status scores for fathers' occupation in Table 67 (which ranged between 37.7 and 53.7, with a concentration in the 40s) indicate that college alumni, whether hearing-impaired or hearing, frequently come from middle-class homes. The mean SEI scores for fathers in the general population range from the high 20s to the low 30s (Blau & Duncan, 1967; Hauser & Featherman, 1977). It is especially interesting to note that both hearing-impaired and hearing females in Samples 1 and 9 had fathers with higher mean SEI scores than the fathers of males in the other six samples. This advantage for hearing-impaired females over hearing-impaired males in Sample 1, however, did not increase their prospects for gains in intergenerational occupational mobility, particularly in respect to obtaining the highest status occupations (80–96 on the SEI scale).

A central conclusion that can be drawn from Table 67 is that almost all samples of respondents have achieved extensive upward occupational mobility over one generation. Mean occupational status scores for all samples of respondents, regardless of hearing ability or gender, were quite a bit higher than their fathers' mean socioeconomic positions. The only exception to this observation was that hearing-impaired males and females educated at NTID had similar mean SEI scores to their fathers. This indicates lack of overall upward occupational mobility for most respondents in this group. More than 80% of these NTID graduates had a vocational diploma, vocational certificate, or an associates degree. Other analyses (Tables 62, 64, 65, and 66) have concluded that acquiring a bachelor's or an advanced degree is a key to opening the door to upward mobility.

Summary

Educational Attainments

Regression analyses of Crammatte's 1983 data (Tables 6–B, 6–C) confirmed prior research results (Schroedel, 1976/1977, 1982b) on the influence of certain attributes of deafness. Attributes such as age at onset, severity of hearing impairment, and quality of speech affected respondents' education more than they influenced respondents' occupational accomplishments.

In regard to age at onset, the postlingually deafened respondents were more likely to have completed advanced degrees than were the prelingually deafened respondents. In regard to speech skills, a larger percentage of good speakers earned postbaccalaureate degrees than did respondents with less than good speech. As a group, the good speakers had a later age at onset of hearing loss and less overall severe hearing impairment. These findings, however, do not obscure the fact that almost 70% of the respondents became deaf before the age of 3, and more than 55% of these respondents have graduate degrees.

Type of college attended for the first degree was also a significant predictor of respondents' educational attainments (Table 6–B). Those from a regular college were found more likely to complete graduate degrees than were respondents who first attended a special college. Differences in characteristics of respondents from each type of undergraduate college help to explain this finding. Those who attended a regular college were less likely to have a profound hearing impairment, and they possessed better overall speech skills than respondents from special colleges. Several factors contribute to understanding the significant relationship between respondents' age and educational attainment. Older respondents were better educated than younger respondents, partially because it takes more time to complete advanced degrees. Additionally, larger proportions of younger respondents were prelingually deafened and less severely hearing impaired than older respondents.

OCCUPATIONAL ATTAINMENTS

Respondents' education is the most statistically significant predictor of their occupational status (Table 6–C). Median Socioeconomic Index scores increased as respondents' level of educational attainment increased. One of the most important factors contributing to the lower occupational status of hearing-impaired females compared to hearing-impaired males was that larger proportions of the women were clustered in teaching and human service jobs. These types of jobs are rated lower on the SEI scale than are the scientific and technological occupations that attracted larger numbers of men. Other relevant factors include (a) males were four times more likely than females to have earned a PhD, (b) males were twice as likely as females to obtain entry into the highest status occupations, and (c) research studies indicate that many deaf youth of both sexes hold traditional attitudes about gender in relationship to social roles and occupations. These attitudes were reflected in the college majors chosen by deaf students in 1974.

The influence of fathers' socioeconomic status on respondents' occupational status was demonstrated by intergenerational mobility patterns. A majority of all respondents of both genders were occupationally upwardly mobile. However, those from lower-class homes experienced more extensive upward mobility than did other respondents; those from upper-class homes were more likely to have encountered downward mobility.

Analysis of Patterns

The overall patterns between these previously discussed relationships are presented in Figure 3. Associations between sociodemographic variables as well as deafness-related variables are displayed as they relate to each other and to respondents' educational and occupational attainments. Fathers' socioeconomic status, in addition to respondents' sex and age, are ascribed statuses evident at respondents' birth. Thus, they may be considered *early factors* influencing respondents' educational and occupational accomplishments. Deafness-related variables may be considered *intermediate factors* in respondents' later socioeconomic attainments.

The arrows in the figure represent the direction of the relationship between two variables. A line with a single arrow indicates that the variable on the left occurs before or predicts the variable on the right. A solid line represents a relatively strong relationship between two variables. A broken line indicates that the relationship between the two variables is relatively weak. These distinctions resulted from the research analyses reported in this chapter.

Several preliminary conclusions can be drawn from Figure 3. One is that disabling effects due to hearing impairment had strong influences on respondents' educational attainment. This is demonstrated by the significant links between (a) age at onset and severity of impairment and (b) speech skills and type of first college attended. It is also evident that the variables that comprise attributes of deafness more

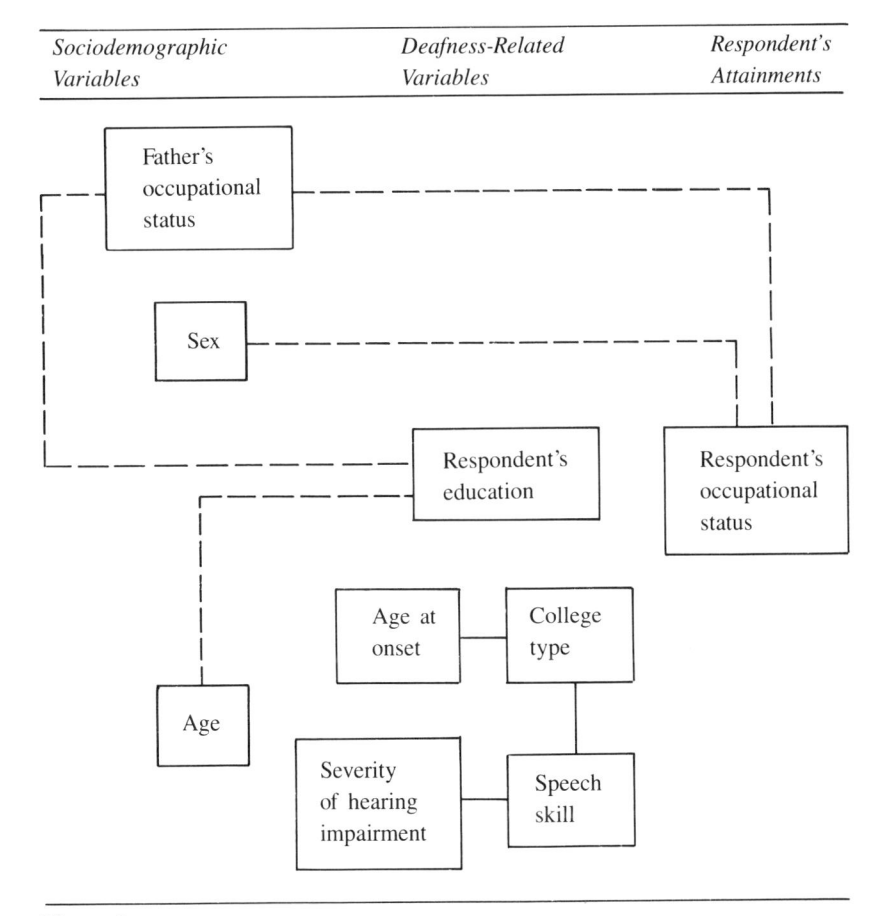

Sociodemographic Variables	Deafness-Related Variables	Respondent's Attainments

Figure 3
Relationships Between Major Variables Influencing Respondents' Educational and Occupational Attainments

strongly influence respondents' educational attainments than they affect respondents' occupationl status. These deafness-related variables create a powerful chain reaction upon consequent variables. Another interesting observation is that respondents' education affects their occupational status more strongly than does their fathers' occupational status. There is also a weak association between fathers' occupation and respondents' education. Taken together, these patterns mean that hearing-impaired respondents can achieve more on the basis of their individual merits than through parental social class. Respondents' gender has a relatively weak but significant influence on respondents' occupational status but not on the other variables in Figure 3.

Several implications from Figure 3 merit discussion. Two of the variables in this figure are modifiable in the sense that they represent a range of options. One of these is type of college. It is desirable that hearing-impaired youth have access to a wide variety of postsecondary programs for their education and vocational training. A key to this success is adequate support services, such as interpreters, tutors, and counselors, in addition to program staff who can communicate with deaf college students. Increasing the variety of educational and occupational training options for hearing-impaired youth may result in an increase in the range of jobs available to hearing-impaired college graduates. The second modifiable variable is respondents' level of education. In order to increase postsecondary educational attainment, hearing-impaired students must improve their abilities to read and write English (Schroedel, 1982b).

Other Results

In comparisons of the socioeconomic attainments of hearing-impaired and hearing persons with a college education, Crammatte's respondents' mean occupational status increased as their level of education increased. However, at comparable levels of education, nearly all samples of hearing respondents had larger mean SEI scores than did hearing-impaired respondents. One of the factors explaining this lack of socioeconomic equality is the underrepresentation of hearing-impaired respondents in high-status professions such as law, medicine, engineering, and dentistry. Continued efforts to improve equal access to high-quality undergraduate and graduate level programs will be a key determinant in whether socioeconomic parity is achieved.

Table 6-A
Matrix of Simple Correlations Between Major Variables

Variable	1	2	3	4	5	6	7	8	9	10
Age										
Sex	−12*									
Fathers' job	−13*	05								
Age at onset	−22*	−03	−12*							
Hearing loss	16*	−01	01	01						
Oral skill	04	07	07	27*	−23*					
First signed	13*	−02	−19*	−10*	10*	−34*				
High school	09	−03	−18*	−20*	17*	−39*	62*			
Education	10*	−01	02	15*	06	12*	−06	−11*		
College type	02	04	09	18*	−15*	28*	−31*	−46*	11*	
Respondents' job	04	−10*	09	02	01	−01	−02	−02	14*	−02

Note. Sign of a correlation between any two coded dichotomous variables (e.g., numbers 2, 7, 8, or 10) or between a coded variable and any other variable is to be interpreted opposite the direction shown. Signs of all other correlations are interpreted as shown. $N=1345$ due to listwise deletion of missing cases. All figures are hundredths; decimals not shown.

*P<.001

Table 6-B
Stepwise Regression Analysis of Major Variables With Respondents' Educational Attainment

Variable	R	R^2	Increase in R^2	F	Beta
Age at Onset	.1504	.0226	.0226	31.12*	.150
Speech Skill	.1737	.0302	.0075	10.45*	.090
Hearing Loss	.1903	.0361	.0061	8.46*	.080
College Type	.2048	.0419	.0057	8.01*	.085
Age	.2135	.0456	.0036	5.10*	.063

Note. The variables list is identical to variables given in Table 6-A with the exception of sector type and respondent's occupational status. The order of entry was computer determined. This program procedure eliminates all variables not shown which do not significantly add to R^2.

*P≤.0001

Table 6-C
Stepwise Regression of Major Variables With
Respondents' Occupational Status

Variable	R	R^2	Increase in R^2	F	Beta
Education	.1425	.0203	.0203	27.85*	.143
Sex	.1735	.0301	.0098	13.57*	−.100
Fathers' Job	.1974	.0390	.0089	18.13*	.094

Note. The variables list is identical to variables given in Table 6-A. The order of entry was computer determined. This program procedure eliminates all variables not shown which do not significantly add to R^2.

*P = .0001

Chapter Seven
COMPARING THE ERAS

In 1960, believing that the capabilities of hearing-impaired adults were being underestimated and overlooked, a study was made to examine the experiences of hearing-impaired persons in professional occupations (Crammatte, 1968). The study group contained hearing-impaired adults who worked in offices and laboratories where daily communication with hearing people was necessary.

Each of the respondents underwent an extensive personal interview that revealed how they came to their occupational choice, what their job-seeking strategies were, and what their on-the-job activities entailed. The interviewer tape recorded the responses; unfortunately, distortions in some of the tapes eliminated 13 of the 100 respondents. The criteria for inclusion in the study group were as follows:
1. The respondent had a severe or profound hearing impairment.
2. The respondent had worked for 3 or more years.
3. The respondent had a minimum salary of $4,000 per year (about $13,000 in 1982 dollars; Bureau of Labor Statistics, 1984).
4. The respondent had a professional or managerial job among co-workers who could hear.

These criteria excluded people who worked with, or for, other hearing-impaired people. They also excluded independent professionals such as dentists, lawyers, doctors.

In order to determine whether hearing-impaired workers had made any progress in professional employment, the 1960 group was compared to a group of hearing-impaired professionals employed in 1982. The criteria for inclusion in the present group were as follows:
1. The respondent had a severe to profound hearing impairment.
2. The respondent had worked for 3 or more years.
3. The respondent had an annual salary of $10,000 or more.
4. The respondent's job was listed as professional or managerial in the 1980 Bureau of the Census list of occupational classifications.
5. The respondent was employed in the hearing sector.

The 1982 group contained 337 hearing-impaired professionals, considerably more than the 1960 study.

COMMUNICATION

The respondents in both the 1960 and 1982 groups had communication skills and problems that were, generally, much more acute than those of people working in the deaf sector. These respondents were all severely or profoundly deaf. They were not, as a rule, able to alleviate the difficulties of oral communication through hearing aids or other devices. They relied on vision for their receptive language ability (e.g., writing, speechreading, or manual means).

Both groups were asked to identify from a list of methods the ones they used most frequently to communicate with hearing co-workers. The methods included writing, talking (and speechreading), sign language, and fingerspelling. Table 69 summarizes the responses into three categories—written, oral, and manual means; manual means include sign language, fingerspelling, and use of an interpreter.

Oral means remained the dominant mode in this employment situation; the change in proportion was not large. There was a significant change in the proportion of workers who used written means: More than one third of the 1960 respondents used written means

Table 69
A Comparison of 1960 and 1982 Respondents' Means of
Communication with Hearing Co-workers
(In %)

	Type of Communication			
	Expressive		Receptive	
Means of Communication	1982 n = 298	1960 n = 87	1982 n = 299	1960 n = 87
Oral	60.4	63	57.5	55
Written	27.5	35	28.8	40
Manual	12.1	2	13.7	5

Note. All data relating to 1960 respondents are from *Deaf Persons in Professional Employment* by A. B. Crammatte, 1968, Springfield, IL: Charles C. Thomas. Copyright 1968 by Charles C. Thomas. Adapted by permission.

compared to a little over one fourth of the 1982 respondents. The use of manual means with hearing co-workers tripled, although only about one eighth of the 1982 respondents used manual means. This latter result may stem from the widespread interest among the general public in learning sign language. Some of this interest may be due to the Communication Skills Program begun by the National Association of the Deaf (NAD) in 1962. Since 1962, the NAD and other groups have provided sign language classes in many states across the country.

Considering the extensive use of oral means by both groups, it is obvious that speech skills are important to the respondents' welfare on the job with hearing co-workers. Table 70 shows how respondents rated their own speech skills.

Recalling the caveats about interpretation of the second level of speech skills in chapter 2, it is appropriate to repeat here the intent of the question. The second level was meant to indicate a level of speech and speechreading that is less than fluent, the ability to carry on a conversation that stumbles and may be strained but does manage to use the oral mode. "A short simple sentence" means a greeting, a brief comment on the weather, or a similar very short statement. The figures in Table 70 show some decline since 1960 in skilled use of speech and a sizable increase in use of speechreading. The totals of the top two expressive scores, however, are very similar in the two periods (about 75%). The 1982 group also scored about 75% for receptive skills, but the 1960 group's scores were only about 63%.

Table 70
A Comparison of Respondents' Speech Skills
(In %)

Speech Skills	Respondents 1982	1960
Expressive	n = 323	n = 84
Co-workers understand:		
Almost all said	38.1	44.0
Almost all said, with care	39.3	34.5
Word or two now and then	15.8	17.9
Respondent does not use speech	6.8	3.6
Receptive	n = 330	n = 87
Respondent understands:		
Almost all said	32.7	20.7
Short conversation, with care	41.2	42.6
Short, simple sentence	16.1	21.8
Word or two now and then	—	12.6
Speech not used to respondent	10.0	2.3

Note. All data relating to 1960 respondents are from *Deaf Persons in Professional Employment* by A. B. Crammatte, 1968, Springfield, IL: Charles C. Thomas. Copyright 1968 by Charles C. Thomas. Adapted by permission.

There is an obvious relationship between use of oral means of communication and a deaf person's speech skills. The data reported in Table 71 demonstrates that the respondents in the 1960 group who used non-oral means of communication had better expressive skills but poorer receptive skills than the respondents in the 1982 group. This can be readily explained by the fact that the proportion of persons deafened later in youth, after learning to talk, was much larger in 1960 than it is today. The reduction of adventitious deafness has come about because of the use of antibiotics with various fevers, more accurate diagnoses, and a marked decrease in infant mortality.

Schroedel (1976/1977) found a larger proportion of younger deaf workers to be prelingually (before age 3) deaf than older deaf workers. This change in age of occurrence of hearing loss has resulted in noticeable differences in communication skills between the two groups of respondents. Persons deafened after age 6 tend to retain speech skills

Table 71
A Comparison of Speech Skills and Means of Communication Used
Most Frequently with Co-workers
(In %)

	Means of Communication			
	1982		1960	
Speech Skills	Oral	Non-Oral	Oral	Non-Oral
Expressive	$n=180$	$n=118$	$n=53$	$n=31$
Co-workers understand:				
Almost all said	59.4	8.5	60.4	16.1
Almost all, with care	40.0	36.5	35.8	32.3
Word or two now and then	0.6	38.2	1.9	45.1
Respondent does not use speech	—	16.8	1.9	6.5
Receptive	$n=172$	$n=127$	$n=43$	$n=39$
Respondent understands:				
Almost all said	50.6	11.8	33.3	5.1
Short conversation, with care	45.3	35.5	56.2	25.6
Short, simple sentence	4.1	29.1	8.3	38.5
Word or two now and then	—	—	—	28.2
Speech not used to respondent	—	23.6	2.2	2.6

Note. All data relating to 1960 respondents are from *Deaf Persons in Professional Employment* by A. B. Crammatte, 1968, Springfield, IL: Charles C. Thomas. Copyright 1968 by Charles C. Thomas. Adapted by permission.

but generally do not become as adept at speechreading as do those deafened before age 6.

Age at onset of deafness also affects choice of communication mode, especially at work (see Table 72). People who have been deafened after they have learned to speak usually prefer to use their speech when communicating with people who hear. They may, however, be poor speechreaders because they have had little practice in developing this skill. Contrastingly, those deafened before age 3 learn to speechread as part of the process of learning to speak, and, therefore, are better speechreaders than the postlingually deaf respondents.

As has already been mentioned, improvements in medicine have radically changed the average age at onset of deafness. Linguists consider age 3 to be the critical age for acquiring a language (Brown, 1973). In the particular group analyzed here (severely and profoundly

Table 72
A Comparison of 1960 and 1982 Respondents' Age of Occurrence
Of Deafness and Their Means of Communication at Work
(In %)

	Means of Communication							
	Expressive				Receptive			
	Oral		Non-Oral		Oral		Non-Oral	
Age of Occurrence	1982	1960	1982	1960	1982	1960	1982	1960
of Deafness	n=181	n=54	n=124	n=32	n=170	n=47	n=131	n=39
Less than 3 years	65.8	42.6	89.5	62.5	73.5	51.1	81.7	48.7
3–5 years	11.6	7.4	7.3	15.6	10.6	10.6	7.6	10.3
6–11 years	11.6	16.7	1.6	21.9	9.4	14.9	4.6	23.1
12 years and over	11.0	33.3	1.6	—	6.5	23.4	6.1	17.9

Note. All data relating to 1960 respondents are from *Deaf Persons in Professional Employment* by A. B. Crammatte, 1968, Springfield, IL: Charles C. Thomas. Copyright 1968 by Charles C. Thomas. Adapted by permission.

deaf adults working in the hearing sector), 80% of the 335 respondents reported losing their hearing before age 3. In each category in Table 72, the proportion of respondents impaired before age 3 is much larger for the 1982 group than for the 1960 group and, conversely, the proportion deafened after age 12 is larger for the 1960 group than for the 1982 group.

Looking at the numbers instead of the percentages, a majority of both groups use oral means of communication for both expressive and receptive language. Table 38 showed that early deafened individuals tended to go into the corporate and government jobs that dominate the hearing sector, and they established themselves as professional workers. Probably this tendency will raise awareness of the capabilities of deaf people by employers and by deaf people themselves.

Age at onset of deafness also affects speech skills. Here the dividing line between easily acquired speech and the intense labors needed to learn it seems to fall at about age 6. Persons who have heard until that age usually have speech and language well enough established to retain it thereafter without too much difficulty. Therefore, they are able to talk relatively fluently (see Table 73). Learning to speechread may be more difficult for the group deafened after age 6. Perhaps the most notable thing about Table 73 is the slightly larger proportions of 1982 respondents who reported having the top speech

Table 73
1960 and 1982 Respondents' Speech Skills by Age of Occurrence of Deafness
(In %)

	Age of Occurrence			
	1982		1960	
Speech Skills	Under 6 Years	6 Years and Over	Under 6 Years	6 Years and Over
Expressive	n = 276	n = 47	n = 49	n = 34
Co-workers understand:				
Almost all said	31.5	76.7	26.5	67.7
Almost all said, with care	42.4	21.2	38.8	29.4
Word or two now and then	18.1	2.1	28.6	2.9
Respondent does not use speech	8.0	—	6.1	—
Receptive	n = 223	n = 49	n = 50	n = 34
Respondent understands:				
Almost all said	32.9	31.9	22.0	17.6
Short conversation, with care	40.2	46.9	36.0	55.9
Short, simple sentence	17.0	10.6	24.0	20.6
Word or two now and then	9.9	10.6	18.0	5.9

Note. All data relating to 1960 respondents are from *Deaf Persons in Professional Employment* by A. B. Crammatte, 1968, Springfield, IL: Charles C. Thomas. Copyright 1968 by Charles C. Thomas. Adapted by permission.

skill compared to the 1960 group. Table 73 also reemphasizes the decreased proportion of adventitiously deafened persons in the deaf population. Only about 17% of the 1982 group were deafened after age 6, whereas close to 40% of the 1960 respondents were deafened after that age.

EDUCATION

As was mentioned in chapter 3, education plays a highly influential role in the professional employment of people with hearing impairments. A high level of educational attainment probably helps to allay uninformed employers' doubts. It also is generally recognized as the chief factor in socioeconomic status.

The number of hearing-impaired students who go on to graduate study has increased markedly in the 22 years between the two studies. In 1960, only 5 out of 87 respondents had earned doctorates; in 1982, 21 out of the 337 respondents employed in the hearing sector had doctorates. There were also 71 other respondents with doctorates from the total group of 1982 respondents (1735). Definitely, much more advanced graduate work is being done by hearing-impaired young people now than was done prior to 1960. Table 74 compares the educational levels of the respondents in both groups. The two groups are divided according to onset of hearing loss before and after age 6. A much greater proportion of the 1982 respondents was graduated from college (80.3%) than were 1960 respondents (70.1%). In both groups a larger proportion of respondents deafened at age 6 or later obtained graduate degrees than did the early deafened respondents. In 1982, the proportion of respondents who had not completed bachelor's degree requirements had declined from almost 30% in 1960 to about 20%.

In examining the situation for deaf students in general colleges and universities, several negative issues become evident, including the problems faced by the deaf students and the adjustments that have to be made in order to cope with an uncongenial environment. In 1960, deaf

Table 74
A Comparison of Respondents' Highest Educational Level Attained with Age When Deafness Occurred
(In %)

Highest Educational Level	1982 Less than Age 6 $n=298$	1982 6 Years and Over $n=35$	1982 Total $n=333$	1960 Less than Age 6 $n=53$	1960 6 Years and Over $n=34$	1960 Total $n=87$
Less than grade 12	0.7	—	0.6	—	—	—
High school graduate	5.0	2.9	4.8	7.5	2.9	5.7
Some college	14.8	5.7	13.8	22.6	26.5	24.3
BA/BS Degree	61.3	14.3	56.5	51.0	35.3	44.8
MA/MS Degree	12.1	45.6	15.6	13.2	29.4	19.5
Three-year Degree	1.7	8.6	2.4	—	—	—
Doctorate	4.4	22.9	6.3	5.7	5.9	5.7

Note. All data relating to 1960 respondents are from *Deaf Persons in Professional Employment* by A. B. Crammatte, 1968, Springfield, IL: Charles C. Thomas. Copyright 1968 by Charles C. Thomas. Adapted by permission.

students who attended a regular college or university were very much on their own. First of all, these institutions were not in the habit of admitting *special students*; therefore, they made the admissions process difficult. Once they admitted special students, they were not prepared for them, and so they failed to provide any support services. Often, professors were insensitive to the special students' needs.

In 1982, 106 colleges and universities offered special help of one kind or another (Rawlings, Karchmer, & DeCaro, 1983). These institutions have placed a great deal of emphasis on providing aids to overcome communication problems. (See chap. 3 for a detailed listing of these aids and the extent of their use).

In the 1960 study, the respondents were asked whether they had attended a school with special programs (i.e., residential school or day school or classes primarily for hearing-impaired students) or a general school without programs for hearing-impaired pupils. The responses were cross-tabulated with data on highest educational level attained by respondents. The type of school listed was the one that the respondent had attended longest. The 1982 questionnaire asked only for the type of high school from which the respondent had graduated. The two categories are not identical; nevertheless, it is of interest to compare these figures (see Table 75).

Table 75
A Comparison of Type of School Respondents Attended and Their Highest Educational Level Attained
(In %)

	Type of School Attended			
	Program for Deaf Students		No Special Program	
Highest Educational Level	1982 $n=178$	1960 $n=55$	1982 $n=153$	1960 $n=32$
Grade 12 or less	3.4	9.1	7.8	—
Some college	15.2	23.6	12.4	24.9
BA/BS Degree	65.1	52.8	45.1	31.3
MA/MS Degree	11.2	12.7	21.6	31.3
Three-year Degree	1.7	—	3.9	—
Doctorate	3.4	1.8	9.2	12.5

Note. All data relating to 1960 respondents are from *Deaf Persons in Professional Employment* by A. B. Crammatte, 1968, Springfield, IL: Charles C. Thomas. Copyright 1968 by Charles C. Thomas. Adapted by permission.

Improvement in educational attainment since 1960 is most marked for graduates of regular schools with programs for hearing-impaired students. This situation may have resulted from increases in the quantity and quality of special higher education for deaf students. Prior to the start of the National Technical Institute for the Deaf in 1969, Gallaudet College offered the only four-year program especially for hearing-impaired students. Gallaudet did not become accredited until 1957. Before 1957, the lack of accreditation contributed greatly to the reluctance of regular colleges and universities to accept the undergraduate credits of Gallaudet College alumni seeking admission to graduate programs. The situation still affects some doctoral applicants.

During the 1960s and 1970s, the deaf community took positive actions to remove the cloak of paternalism that had been smothering them for the past century. The improved environment was another element that probably encouraged the 1982 respondents to pursue graduate study. Section 504 of the Rehabilitation Act of 1973 was used to enforce their demands. One case, *Davis v. Southeastern Community College* (Crammatte, 1979), was carried to the Supreme Court.

Another factor that helped push many hearing-impaired teachers into graduate study was stricter enforcement of teacher certifying standards by the states. However, that condition must have had only an indirect influence on respondents who worked in the hearing sector; only two of the respondents employed in the hearing sector were teachers. In both periods, 1960 and 1982, graduate study had been undertaken by a greater proportion of respondents from schools with no special programs (43.8% in 1960 and 34.7% in 1982) than of respondents from schools with programs for hearing-impaired students (14.5% in 1960 and 16.3% in 1982).

The data obtained from the respondents was also used to compare the highest level of education attained by graduates from colleges primarily serving deaf students (Gallaudet; NTID/RIT; and California State University, Northridge) and colleges primarily for hearing students (Table 76). A majority (53%) of the 1982 graduates from general colleges obtained graduate degrees, compared to 46.7% of the 1960 group. The tendency of graduates of regular colleges to go on to higher professional training might be explained in part by (a) their familiarity with the environment and (b) the influence of a mentor who encouraged more professional preparation.

Table 76
Relationship Between Type of College Respondents Attended and
Their Highest Educational Level Attained
(In %)

Highest Educational Level	Respondents			
	Special Colleges		General Colleges	
	1982 $n=191$	1960 $n=31$	1982 $n=83$	1960 $n=30$
No degree	0.5	—	3.6	—
BA/BS Degree	79.0	74.2	43.4	53.3
MA/MS Degree	15.7	25.8	27.7	30.0
Three-year Degree	1.6	—	7.2	—
Doctorate	3.2	—	18.1	16.7

Note. All data relating to 1960 respondents are from *Deaf Persons in Professional Employment* by A. B. Crammatte, 1968, Springfield, IL: Charles C. Thomas. Copyright 1968 by Charles C. Thomas. Adapted by permission.

Looking at the numerical data in Tables 75 and 76, it can be seen that a fairly large group of the 1982 respondents, 153 (46.2%), were graduated from high schools with no special program for deaf students. Only 83 (30.3%) were baccalaureate graduates of general colleges and universities. In 1960, 32 (36.8%) of the respondents were graduated from high schools with no special program, but almost half earned their bachelor's degree at general colleges. This change may due be to the special colleges' efforts to become accredited, offer more major areas of study, and publicize their programs more effectively.

The 1960 study did not include workers in the deaf sector. Therefore, no directly comparable data is available. Since, in 1960, teachers comprised more than 90% of professional workers in this sector, the only comparable employment data in the deaf sector in 1960 is for educators of deaf students. In 1960, the number of *deaf* teachers (actually deaf and hard of hearing) reported in the *American Annals of the Deaf* was 477 (Doctor, 1961). For 1982, the figure is 1,268 (Craig & Craig, 1983). For the same period, the total number of teachers of hearing-impaired students in the United States grew from 4,100 in 1960 to 8,053 in 1982.

Among all teachers in schools and classes for hearing-impaired students in the United States in both 1960 and 1982, deaf teachers made up 11.6%. However, a notable difference for hearing-impaired educators in 1982 was their upward mobility. Comparable data are not available, but close observation of the conditions in 1960 shows no deaf employees who were school superintendents, less than a dozen principals, and even fewer clinical personnel. The present study shows that 141 respondents held managerial positions (three were residential school superintendents), 102 were management-related employees, 16 were social scientists, 33 were social and recreational workers, 23 were librarians and archivists, and 130 were educational and vocational counselors (not dormitory counselors). Not all, but certainly a huge majority, of these respondents worked in schools for deaf students.

It seems apparent that there has been an upgrading of quality and quantity of professional positions in the deaf sector. However, if this upgrading is taken into account, then the proportion of deaf educational staff has declined in schools and classes in the United States. The total educational staff (administrators, teachers, full-time teacher aides, clinical personnel, and media and library workers) has risen from 4,440 in 1960 to 14,496 in 1982. Taking educational staff (not just teachers) as the basis for calculation, the proportion of deaf workers to the the total was 10.8% in 1960 and 8.7% in 1982.

Fathers' occupation affects family status, which in turn affects a child's educational expectations and attainment (Jencks et al., 1979; Schroedel, 1976/1977). The 1960 study cross-classified educational attainment with father's occupation. Jobs were classified as either white-collar (management, professional specialty, technical, sales, or administrative) or blue-collar (service, crafts, industrial production, farming). Table 77 compares the findings for 1960 and 1982.

The two groups of respondents from white-collar families had fairly equal educational attainment levels. A somewhat larger proportion of the 1982 respondents had earned college degrees but, interestingly, a slightly larger proportion of the 1960 respondents had earned graduate degrees. The 1982 group of respondents from blue-collar families was better educated than the 1960 group. This was especially notable at the graduate level. From another point of view, Table 77 shows 129 of 321 (40.2%) respondents in the 1982 group had moved from blue-collar families into professional employment. Similarly, 30 of the 84 (35.7%) 1960 respondents came from blue-collar families.

Table 77
Relationship Between Respondents' Highest Level of Education
And Their Fathers' Occupations
(In %)

	Father's Occupation			
	White Collar		Blue Collar	
Highest Educational	1982	1960	1982	1960
Level Attained	n = 192	n = 54	n = 129	n = 30
Less than BA/BS Degree	19.3	24.1	20.9	40.0
BA/BS Degree	53.1	42.6	58.2	50.0
Graduate study	27.6	33.3	20.9	10.0

Note. All data relating to 1960 respondents are from *Deaf Persons in Professional Employment* by A. B. Crammatte, 1968, Springfield, IL: Charles C. Thomas. Copyright 1968 by Charles C. Thomas. Adapted by permission.

Apparently, the *American Dream* of upward mobility has come true for a larger proportion of the deaf population since 1960. Certainly, there have been complaints of high unemployment in the past, and they continue today. Yet, the socioeconomic status of some of the survey respondents is higher than that of their parents.

Is an advanced degree a key to higher earnings? The consistently rising median salary for each college degree (Table 78) seems to answer this question insofar as the 1982 respondents are concerned. Indeed, the holders of doctoral degrees report a median salary almost double that of those with no degree.

The 1960 data can be made comparable to those of 1982 by converting 1960 dollars into 1982 dollars. The conversion formula (3.253664) comes from the Consumer Price Index (Bureau of Labor Statistics, 1984). The median salary reported in 1960 was $7,576. This is equivalent to about $24,650 1982 dollars, which is somewhat less than the $26,291 reported in 1982.

The 1960 data are insufficient for computing reliable medians at various educational levels of the respondents. However, of those who had graduate degrees, 63.6% earned more than the top of the median class ($26,000). Only 38.5% of those with bachelor's degrees earned above the median class interval.

Another approach to answering the question of whether advanced educational training yields higher returns in salary is to examine the proportions of respondents who earn more than the median income of

Table 78
A Comparison of 1982 Respondents Annual Salaries and
Their Highest Level of Education
(In %)

	Highest Educational Degree				
Salary	No Degree	Bachelor's Degree	Graduate Degree	Doctorate	Total
Under $10,000	—	4	—	—	4
$10,000–$14,999	5	12	2	—	19
$15,000–$19,999	22	31	8	1	62
$20,000–$24,999	15	39	8	1	63
$25,000–$29,999	10	39	10	1	60
$30,000–$34,999	5	26	10	2	43
$35,000–$39,999	1	20	10	4	35
$40,000–$44,999	1	9	3	5	18
$45,000–$49,999	—	2	4	—	6
$50,000 and over	2	2	6	7	17
Total	61	184	61	21	327
Median salaries	$21,166	$25,769	$31,250	$41,500	$26,291

the total group (see Table 79). The proportions of those earning higher than average salaries varies greatly for the two groups—from 31.3% of those 1982 workers with no degree to 90.5% of those with a doctorate. The 1960 figures vary similarly from 34.6% to 80%, respectively, for these two categories. The percentage of respondents earning above average salaries is greater at each level of educational attainment.

It is quite evident that in both periods the higher the educational degree attained the more the individual should be earning. These data ignore other variables such as the respondent's age and years of service. The fact that larger proportions of persons with bachelor's and master's degrees from the 1982 group earned better than average salaries probably results from better specialized higher education opportunities for deaf people and stiffer expectations from employers.

OCCUPATIONS AND ECONOMIC CONDITIONS

The main assumption made in planning the present study was that the number and variety of deaf professional workers increased significantly

Table 79
Proportions of Respondents' Salaries Above Approximate Medians
When Compared with Their Highest Level of Education

	Respondents			
	1982		1960	
	$25,000 and over		$26,000 and over	
Highest Educational Level	Number	Percent	Number	Percent
No degree	20/64	31.3	9/26	34.6
BA/BS Degree	98/185	53.0	15/39	38.5
MA/MS Degree	36/57	63.2	10/17	58.8
Three-year Degree	8/10	80.0	—	—
Doctorate	19/21	90.5	4/5	80.0

Note. All data relating to 1960 respondents are from *Deaf Persons in Professional Employment* by A. B. Crammatte, 1968, Springfield, IL: Charles C. Thomas. Copyright 1968 by Charles C. Thomas. Adapted by permission. The median salary for the 1982 group was $26,291. The median for 1960 was $7,576, which lies in the upper area of the class interval $6,000–7,999. It is not possible to retrieve details of individual salaries within the class intervals of 1960; therefore, for comparison purposes, the nearest class limit is used here and in subsequent analyses. This treatment results in levels of comparison of $26,000 for 1960 and $25,000 for 1982. The Consumer Price Index shows a conversion ratio for 1960 to 1982 dollars of 3.253664.

in the period between 1960 and 1982. That assumption was examined using the narrow interpretation of *deaf*. The respondents analyzed in this chapter all reported themselves as severely or profoundly deaf (see Appendix B for an explanation of terms). Table 80 lists the various occupational categories covering the positions held by respondents in 1960 and 1982.

Among the more notable occupational differences between the two groups were the many 1982 respondents in management or management-related positions (93 in 1982/5 in 1960). Most management-related workers were accountants (4 of 5 in 1960/50 of 93 in 1982). Another area of difference was the number of respondents holding computer-related jobs—86 of the 1982 respondents were employed as computer analysts or programmers, 7 were operations analysts, 2 were statisticians, and 8 were mathematical scientists. (See Appendix E for detailed data on occupations.)

Another notable difference between the 1960 and 1982 groups is the large number of technicians reported in 1982. In the past, it seemed that almost all deaf people had to prove their worth at lower levels

Table 80
Breakdown of Respondents' Occupational Categories by Gender

| | \multicolumn{6}{c}{Respondents} |
| Occupational Categories | \multicolumn{3}{c}{1982} | \multicolumn{3}{c}{1960} |
	Male	Female	Total	Male	Female	Total
Executive, administrative, and managerial occupations	29	5	34	1	—	1
Management-related occupations	43	16	59	3	1	4
Professional specialty jobs						
Architects	4	1	5	1	—	1
Engineers, Surveyors, and Mapping Scientists	24	—	24	19	—	19
Mathematicians and Computer Scientists	54	8	62	8	1	9
Natural Scientists	23	1	24	30	—	30
Health diagnosing occupations	5	—	5	—	—	—
Health assessment and treating occupations	—	4	4	—	—	—
Teachers, postsecondary	—	1	1	—	—	—
Teachers, except postsecondary	—	2	2	—	—	—
Counselors, educational and vocational	—	1	1	—	—	—
Librarians, Archivists, and Curators	5	4	9	1	4	5
Social Scientists	3	—	3	—	—	—
Social and Recreational Workers	1	—	1	1	—	1
Lawyers and Judges	5	1	6	1	—	1
Writers, Artists, Entertainers, and Athletes	5	3	8	3	2	5
Technicians and support workers						
Health Technologists and Technicians	8	15	23	1	—	1
Engineering Technologists and Technicians	17	1	18	10	—	10
Science Technicians, biological	—	1	1	—	—	—
Other Technicians	34	13	47	—	—	—
Total	260	77	337	79	8	87

Note. All data relating to 1960 respondents are from *Deaf Persons in Professional Employment* by A. B. Crammatte, 1968, Springfield, IL: Charles C. Thomas. Copyright 1968 by Charles C. Thomas. Adapted by permission.

before they were accepted in the ranks of professional workers. Employers now are apparently more willing to suspend doubts and hire young deaf people on the basis of their education. The technicians in the 1982 group were of a fairly high level. A number of technicians with short tenure and/or low salaries were excluded from the research group on grounds that they had not yet proven their professional potential.

Both groups were heavily involved in the sciences—almost 80% of the 1960 respondents and about 36% of the 1982 respondents. The 1982 group was engaged in a greater variety of occupations; workers held jobs in each of the categories listed in Table 80. In 1960, respondents were not employed in eight of the occupations, and only one respondent was employed in each of five occupations. Of the individual occupations (Appendix E), the 1982 respondents were represented in 41 compared to 28 for 1960 respondents.

A significant difference appears in the proportion of deaf women who held professional/managerial jobs in 1982. Women accounted for almost 25% of the 1982 group compared to only 10% of the 1960 group. Barnartt and Christiansen (1985) noted a big change in deaf women's employment. Their data showed that the percentage of deaf women in blue-collar jobs declined from 51.1% in 1972 to 39.7% in 1977. In the same period, employment of deaf women rose from 37.3% to 41.6% in white-collar jobs and from 11.5% to 19.1% in pink-collar jobs. In 1920, 8% of deaf women held pink-collar jobs and only 4% held white-collar jobs. The implication of upward movement for women contained in the present study is limited considerably by the fact that 30 of the 77 women were technicians, a job classification that is lower on the status scale than either managers or professional specialists.

The percentage of prelingually deaf (before age 3) respondents increased from 49.4% of the 1960 group to 76.3% of the 1982 group. In every occupational category, except the executive group, more than half of the 1982 workers were deafened before age 3 (Table 81). Overall, 63.3% of the group had been deafened before age 1, including, of course, those who were born deaf. The point to remember in this regard is that those who were deafened early acquired language skills the hardest possible way. They did not have the benefit of

Table 81
Respondents' Occupational Categories and
Their Age When Deafness Occurred
(In %)

Occupational Categories	Number of Respondents	Age of Occurrence of Deafness			
		Less than 3 Years	3–5 Years	6–11 Years	12 Years and Over
Executive, administrative, and managerial occupations	34	47.1	14.7	14.7	23.5
Management-related occupations	60	84.8	8.5	5.0	1.7
Professional specialty workers					
Architects	5	60.0	40.0	—	—
Engineers, Surveyors, and Mapping Scientists	24	75.1	12.5	4.1	8.3
Mathematicians and Computer Scientists	62	71.0	17.7	11.3	—
Natural Scientists	24	70.9	8.3	8.3	12.5
Health diagnosing workers	5	60.0	20.0	—	20.0
Health assessment and treating occupations	4	100.0	—	—	—
Teachers, postsecondary	1	100.0	—	—	—
Teachers, except postsecondary	2	50.0	—	—	50.0
Counselors, educational and vocational	1	—	100.0	—	—
Librarians, Archivists, and Curators	8	87.5	12.5	—	—
Social Scientists	2	—	50.0	—	50.0
Social and Recreational Workers	1	100.0	—	—	—
Lawyers and Judges	5	60.0	—	—	40.0
Writers, Artists, Entertainers, and Athletes	8	100.0	—	—	—
Technicians and support jobs					
Health Technologists and Technicians	23	82.7	—	13.0	4.3
Engineering Technologists and Technicians	18	83.3	11.1	5.6	—
Science Technicians, biological	1	—	—	—	100.0
Other Technicians	47	93.7	2.1	2.1	2.1
All Categories	335	76.3	9.6	7.2	6.9

auditory stimuli surrounding them all their waking hours. They had to learn each word and polish their reading and writing skills by conscious effort. On top of this, some may have had to contend with the reaction of an unknowing employer or co-worker who was not comfortable with a person so different.

In 1960, speech skills were examined in relation to occupational categories (Table 82). Lunde and Bigman (1959) had found speechreading ability to be related to occupational level. Sixty of the 1960 respondents stated that absence of a need for frequent oral communication was an outstanding characteristic of an occupation suitable for deaf persons. Of these 60 respondents, 46 were employed in the natural sciences and mathematics. These results lead one to ask whether deaf people with less than maximum speech skills make a conscious decision to enter those professions in the hearing sector that are laboratory- or workroom-oriented rather than those that are people-oriented. However, more research is needed before this question can be answered.

Table 82
A Comparison of Speech Skills of Respondents in
Scientific and Other Occupations
(In %)

	1982		1960	
Speech Skills	Scientists $n=125$	Other $n=205$	Scientists $n=64$	Other $n=23$
Expressive				
Top skill	29.6	44.9	40.7	47.8
Next level	41.6	37.1	35.9	26.1
All other levels	28.8	18.0	23.4	26.1
Receptive				
Top skill	26.2	36.9	15.6	34.8
Next level	45.2	38.8	42.2	43.5
All other levels	28.6	24.3	42.2	21.7

Note. All data relating to 1960 respondents are from *Deaf Persons in Professional Employment* by A. B. Crammatte, 1968, Springfield, IL: Charles C. Thomas. Copyright 1968 by Charles C. Thomas. Adapted by permission. Top speech skill denotes ability to speak or speechread almost all said; the next level indicates ability to speak so as to be understood but needing frequent repetitions or the ability to speechread only a short conversation.

It is difficult to determine comparable median salaries for these groups. The closest feasible approximations (figured in 1982 dollars) were $26,000 for 1960 and $25,000 for 1982. The calculation of these figures, using the Consumer Price Index ratio for the conversion rate, was noted in Table 79.

Both eras reflect similar relationships of salary to age. The largest proportions of lower salaries went to respondents below age 35. Similarly, the larger salaries were paid mainly to respondents between the ages of 35 and 54. The modal class for the 1982 group was ages 35–44; for 1960, it was 45–54 (see Table 83).

Comparison of the higher salaried groups for the two periods arouses some speculation. The proportion of 1982 respondents below age 45 who earned higher salaries (65.2%) was considerably larger than the under-45 group of 1960 respondents (44.7%). This earlier climb to better salaries for younger 1982 respondents may be a reflection of the improved educational opportunities they have enjoyed. More of them were graduated from college (80.3% compared to 70.1% of the 1960 group). Also, the quality and variety of course offerings became much greater in specialized colleges for hearing-impaired students during the 1960s and 1970s than they had been before 1960. Other factors to consider are the improvement of placement services for

Table 83
A Comparison of Respondents' Salaries by Age
(In %)

	\multicolumn{2}{c}{Salaries}		
	\multicolumn{2}{c}{1982}	\multicolumn{2}{c}{1960}
Age in Years	Under $25,000 n=148	$25,000 and Over n=181	Under $26,000 n=49	$26,000 and Over n=38
Below 35	54.7	18.8	34.7	10.5
35–44	29.1	46.4	24.5	34.2
45–54	8.8	21.0	20.4	44.8
55 and over	7.4	13.8	20.4	10.5

Note. All data relating to 1960 respondents are from *Deaf Persons in Professional Employment* by A. B. Crammatte, 1968, Springfield, IL: Charles C. Thomas. Copyright 1968 by Charles C. Thomas. Adapted by permission.

hearing-impaired college graduates and a more accepting attitude by some employers.

As has been noted in previous chapters, marked differences existed in both groups between the salaries earned by hearing-impaired men and women. In 1960, all eight of the women respondents earned less than the $26,000 median salary. In 1982, conditions were slightly improved; 82.6% of the women in the group earned less than $25,000. Almost 66% of the 1982 male respondents earned salaries higher than $25,000, while 48.1% of the 1960 group earned above $26,000.

Table 84 breaks down salaries by occupational categories. This table shows that in nine occupations, more than half of the 1982 respondents earned salaries higher than the median ($25,000). This group included executives, engineers, mathematicians, natural scientists, health diagnosticians, librarians, architects, and lawyers. Of the 1960 respondents, the data show higher salaries only for executives, engineers, and lawyers. The data are biased in that the $25,000 dividing point for 1982 is about $1,000 less than the actual median, and the 1960 dividing point is about $1,500 more than the median. Lacking raw data for 1960, a closer approximation is not possible.

In both eras and in both salary ranges, a majority of deaf workers employed in the hearing sector adapted to the prevailing oral communication mode. Table 85 shows that the proportion of orally communicating respondents was greatest in the higher salary jobs, especially for expressive communication (71.1% of the 1960 group). One notable change from 1960 was an increase in the use of manual communication by the 1982 respondents at both salary levels. This change may reflect the growth in the number of sign language classes for the public.

Most of the respondents earning above average salaries in both periods had top expressive speech skills (see Table 86). Their receptive skills were not as high; most reported the ability to understand a short, carefully spoken conversation. The proportion of respondents who did not use speech for expression remained about the same; the respondents in 1960 did not indicate nonuse of speech for reception. The proportion of higher paid 1960 respondents able to speak at least fairly well was high (91.7%), probably because a high percentage of them were deafened after age 6.

Table 84
Respondents' Occupational Categories and Salaries Above and Below Median Class Intervals
(In %)

Occupational Categories	Salary Levels					
	1982			1960		
	Number of Respondents	Under $25,000	$25,000 and Over	Number of Respondents	Under $26,000	$26,000 and Over
Executive, administrative, and managerial jobs	32	21.9	78.1	1	—	100.0
Management-related occupations	60	56.7	43.3	4	75.0	25.0
Professional specialty workers						
Architects	5	40.0	60.0	1	100.0	—
Engineers, Surveyors, and Mapping Scientists	23	13.0	87.0	19	21.1	78.9
Mathematicians and Computer Scientists	60	36.7	63.3	9	66.7	33.3
Natural Scientists	24	20.8	79.2	30	56.7	43.3
Health diagnosing occupations	5	20.0	80.0	—	—	—
Health assessment and treating occupations	4	100.0	—	—	—	—
Teachers, postsecondary	1	100.0	—	—	—	—
Teachers, except postsecondary	2	50.0	50.0	—	—	—
Counselors, educational and vocational	1	100.0	—	—	—	—
Librarians, Archivists, and Curators	9	44.4	55.6	5	100.0	—
Social Scientists	2	—	100.0	—	—	—
Social and Recreational Workers	1	100.0	—	1	—	100.0
Lawyers and Judges	6	—	100.0	1	—	100.0
Writers, Artists, Entertainers, and Athletes	7	85.7	14.3	5	60.0	40.0
Technicians and support workers						
Health Technologists and Technicians	22	95.5	4.5	1	100.0	—

Table 84 *(continued)*

	Salary Levels					
	1982			1960		
Occupational Categories	Number of Respondents	Under $25,000	$25,000 and Over	Number of Respondents	Under $26,000	$26,000 and Over
Engineering Technologists and Technicians	17	64.7	35.3	10	100.0	—
Science Technicians, biological	1	100.0	—	—	—	—
Other Technicians	47	51.1	48.9	—	—	—
All Categories	329	45.0	55.0	87	56.3	43.7

Note. All data relating to 1960 respondents are from *Deaf Persons in Professional Employment* by A. B. Crammatte, 1968, Springfield, IL: Charles C. Thomas. Copyright 1968 by Charles C. Thomas. Adapted by permission.

Table 85
A Comparison of Respondents' Salaries with Their Means of Communication with Hearing Co-Workers
(In %)

	Salaries			
	1982		1960	
Means of Communication	Under $25,000	$25,000 and Over	Under $26,000	$26,000 and Over
Expressive	n = 131	n = 168	n = 49	n = 38
Oral	51.2	66.7	57.1	71.1
Written	33.5	23.2	38.8	28.9
Manual	15.3	10.1	4.1	—
Receptive	n = 135	n = 161	n = 49	n = 38
Oral	50.4	62.1	53.1	57.8
Written	33.3	26.1	42.8	36.9
Manual	16.3	11.8	4.1	5.3

Note. All data relating to 1960 respondents are from *Deaf Persons in Professional Employment* by A. B. Crammatte, 1968, Springfield, IL: Charles C. Thomas. Copyright 1968 by Charles C. Thomas. Adapted by permission.

Table 86
Respondents' Salaries and Speech Skills
(In %)

	Salaries			
	1982		1960	
Speech Skills	Under $25,000	$25,000 and Over	Under $26,000	$26,000 and Over
Expressive	n=142	n=175	n=48	n=36
Co-workers understand:				
Almost all said	32.4	43.4	33.3	55.6
Almost all, with care	43.6	36.0	31.3	36.1
Word or two now and then	14.8	16.0	27.1	5.5
Respondent does not use speech	9.2	4.6	8.3	2.8
Receptive	n=146	n=178	n=47	n=35
Respondent understands:				
Almost all said	34.8	31.5	19.1	24.3
Short conversation with care	37.1	44.9	42.6	42.8
Short, simple sentence	12.3	—	17.0	8.6
Word or two, now and then	15.8	15.2	21.3	24.3
Speech not used to respondent	—	8.4	—	—

Note. All data relating to 1960 respondents are from *Deaf Persons in Professional Employment* by A. B. Crammatte, 1968, Springfield, IL: Charles C. Thomas. Copyright 1968 by Charles C. Thomas. Adapted by permission.

ON-THE-JOB PROBLEMS

It is probably true that the deaf person with better speech skills has an advantage at work. It is easier for him or her to socialize, discuss work problems, and join the grapevine. Also, co-workers experience less frustration about their own inability to communicate. However, there are deaf persons who do not speak at all and overcome communication difficulties through their expansive, outgoing personalities.

The 1960 respondents revealed three major communication problems on the job—the telephone, group conferences, and dealing with strangers for the first time. However, they offered solutions to these problems. Some respondents had trained their secretaries to assist on the telephone via sign language, writing, or careful speech. Likewise, secretaries and co-workers helped at conferences. Some organizations provided an agenda prior to staff meetings or a summary afterwards. In dealing with strangers, many respondents mentioned the problem of making the stranger feel at ease.

The 1982 questionnaire asked respondents to check and evaluate a number of communication aids. Their responses are found in Table 87. The most helpful aid was a co-worker who would take notes at meetings or make telephone calls. These respondents rarely used a hearing aid or a telephone amplifier, probably because most were severely or profoundly deaf.

Two of the more effective aids were telecommunication devices for deaf people (TDDs) and trained professional interpreters. TDDs make it possible for a deaf person to have direct telephone contact with the person he or she is calling. However, there is a limitation in that the person receiving the call must have a similar device. The number of business firms and government agencies installing TDDs for consumers has been growing as deaf awareness has increased. Some employers with more than one deaf worker have provided TDDs for internal use.

Professional interpreters are a boon for ease of communication, and they are trained to be unobtrusive. It may be very difficult to justify the cost of an interpreter for a single deaf worker. Sometimes the solution to this problem is a job position with dual responsibility, for example, a secretary/interpreter.

Table 87
Respondents' Rating of Communication Aids
(In %)

Aids to Communication	Number of Responses	Very Helpful	Fairly Helpful	Not Helpful	Do Not Have
TDD	316	46.2	10.4	7.0	36.4
Interpreter	311	41.5	10.3	1.3	46.9
Telephone amplifier	299	9.4	5.7	14.4	70.5
Hearing aid	304	22.7	11.2	15.5	50.6
Secretary[a]	311	37.3	19.3	5.1	38.3
Co-worker[a]	309	48.2	31.3	2.9	17.6
Agenda before meeting	300	31.7	24.0	8.7	35.6
Summary after meeting	300	39.0	33.3	6.7	21.0

[a]Used as a notetaker and/or telephone assistant

As part of the 1960 survey, respondents' colleagues were asked to rate the respondents' effectiveness on the job as compared to that of hearing peers. These colleagues, of all ranks from CEO to receptionist, rated the deaf workers as doing better than their peers in 64.4% of the cases; another 25.3% said respondents were doing as well as their peers. Since no colleagues were interviewed in 1982, the only comparison possible was with the percentage of respondents who had received promotions or awards. Promotions were granted to 67.4% of the respondents; 28.6% of those receiving promotions had been given four or more. Merit awards were made to 68.5% of the respondents.

In order to determine whether these professionals had experienced job discrimination, the 1982 group was asked, "How often have you experienced unfair rejection by employers in each of the job activities listed below?" The results are shown in Table 88. In 1960 the question was, "Has a job, a promotion, or a chance to present your ideas ever been denied you because of your deafness?"

A comparison of the 1960 and 1982 situations can be achieved by examining the proportion of *nevers*. In 1960, 64.7% of those responding said they had not experienced discrimination; in 1982, more than 50% of the responses were *never* or *almost never* for all situations except communication. In regard to communication, 54.9% of the 1982 respondents perceived unfair rejection at least sometimes. The categories *often* and *very often* were cited by 17.5% of the respondents in the case of hiring and by 16.5% in the case of promotion.

Table 88
Perceived Discrimination by Frequency of the Experience
(In %)

Employment Area	Number of Responses	Very Often	Often	Sometimes	Almost Never	Never
Hiring	308	7.8	9.7	23.4	18.2	40.9
Promotion	309	5.8	10.7	28.8	23.3	31.4
Training on the job	314	4.1	8.0	19.4	22.3	46.2
Work evaluation	312	3.2	6.7	22.8	21.5	45.8
Communication	315	7.3	5.4	42.2	20.3	24.8
Salary	312	3.5	6.4	24.4	23.4	42.3

Another way of looking at a job is in terms of job satisfaction. Respondents in 1982 were asked how well they liked or disliked certain aspects of their jobs. Table 89 sums up their responses. Respondents working in the deaf sector enjoyed somewhat higher satisfaction in all respects except promotion and salary. Promotions were rare among teachers and salaries were notoriously low in human services jobs. Unfortunately, most of the deaf sector workers were employed in these two areas. The total index of job satisfaction for the 1982 group was 1.27 compared to 1.21 for the deaf sector. Both figures denote rather high satisfaction; 2.0 is the top score, -2 the score for complete dissatisfaction.

The 1960 respondents were not asked about job satisfaction directly, they were asked about life aspirations. Thirty-four out of 75 respondents related "the best way of life" to their work situations. Also, the 89.7% of the same group who were rated by colleagues as being as good or better than co-workers in similar positions were often described as being "keen for their work."

Summary

Deaf professional workers in the hearing sector in 1982 found a larger proportion of co-workers able to communicate with them by manual

Table 89
Respondents' Rating of Job Satisfaction
(In %)

Extent of Liking	Chances for Promotion $n=315$	Kind of Work $n=325$	Supervisors $n=319$	Colleagues $n=319$	Subordinates $n=313$	Salary $n=320$
Like very much	47.7	74.2	58.4	64.3	46.6	50.3
Like a little	22.2	17.8	26.0	27.3	15.7	35.0
Dislike a little	5.1	5.5	7.5	2.2	1.9	9.4
Dislike very much	4.7	2.2	2.5	0.6	1.6	4.4
Does not apply	20.3	0.3	5.6	5.6	34.2	0.9
Index of job satisfaction						
1982 subgroup	1.03	1.56	1.30	1.52	1.04	1.18
Deaf sector[a]	0.71	1.69	1.34	1.65	1.11	0.75

[a]From pp. 13–16; see Appendix F for explanation of indexes.

means than did the 1960 group. A majority in both periods, however, adapted to an oral work environment by using oral communication, and most were fairly proficient. Those respondents deafened after age 6 were, by a large majority, proficient with speech but less so with speechreading. This was especially true for the 1960 group. Age of occurrence among the 1982 respondents was generally before age 6. These respondents were more adept at speechreading than at speech. Levels of educational attainment were much higher among the 1982 respondents than among the 1960 respondents. College degrees were received by 80.8% of the 1982 respondents compared to 70.1% in 1960. Doctorates were earned by 6.3% of the 1982 respondents compared to 5.7% of the 1960 group. These advances in education probably arose from higher quality and variety in educational opportunities at specialized colleges (Gallaudet, NTID/RIT, and CSUN) and provision of support services at an increasing number of other colleges and universities. A larger proportion of graduates from general colleges advanced to higher degrees than graduates from specialized colleges. The higher the degree attained, the higher the median salary earned.

The 1982 group of respondents held a greater variety of occupations than did the 1960 group (54 compared to 28). In 1960 the concentration of occupations was in chemistry and engineering; in 1982 the concentration was in executive and management-related positions and in the sciences (especially mathematics and computer science).

The proportion of deaf women in these professional positions in 1982 was much higher than in 1960 (25% compared to 10%). However, women's salaries were lower than men's in both groups. Age of occurrence of deafness was much earlier among the 1982 respondents than it was among the 1960 respondents. With respect to salary, the 1982 group was a little better off, the median salary exceeded that of 1960 by about $1,600 per year in 1982 dollars. The higher the salary, the greater the tendency for workers to use oral communication.

Telecommunication devices for deaf people and interpreters are new and helpful aids to deaf people at work. The most frequent help, though, still comes from friendly co-workers. Discrimination has rarely been experienced by these workers; a majority in both groups reported having never or almost never perceived unfair rejection. In 1982 workers had an index of job satisfaction of 1.27, which means they liked all aspects of their jobs more than a little.

Chapter Eight
PERSPECTIVES ON EMPLOYMENT

Steven L. Jamison

Automation, education, and attitudes are three of the most significant factors that influence the employment patterns of deaf people. Specifically, expanding levels of automation in the office and in the factory, low levels of educational preparation by deaf job seekers, and poor attitudes toward deaf applicants by business and industry have all contributed in the past to the underemployment so characteristic of the deaf population. But the picture is changing.

Computers and robotics are accelerating the pace of automation, yet increasing numbers of deaf students are taking advantage of the new educational alternatives available to them. As a result, employers' attitudes toward deaf workers have markedly improved. Consequently, more and more deaf individuals are employed in positions that will allow the realization of career potentials.

> The 1960 study included information derived from short interviews with hearing colleagues of the respondents. For the 1982 study, time and funds did not permit the interview approach, so information on attitudes of co-workers toward deaf employees was lacking. In its place Dr. Steven L. Jamison was asked to contribute a chapter on employment prospects. As a long-time personnel consultant with IBM and the father of a hearing-impaired son, Dr. Jamison has been an effective advocate for employment of hearing-impaired professionals in business.

AUTOMATION

Much has been said about the effect of automation and the consequent elimination of many low-level jobs. However, the trend toward increased automation shows no signs of slowing down, nor should it for two very important reasons—
1. Internally, the soundness of our economy requires constant searching for ways to increase productivity. This can be done by individuals working harder or working smarter. Traditionally, we have preferred working smarter (i.e., using machines to greatly expand the productivity of individuals).
2. Externally, the United States is losing its competitive edge in world markets. "Yankee know-how" is becoming "Yankee knew-how" in the face of highly innovative developments in countries such as Japan and West Germany. All of this seems to encourage more widespread and more sophisticated office automation and industrial robotics for the future.

Although, for a fixed level of production, automation sometimes implies an increase in the number of higher-level jobs, it nearly always implies an even greater decrease in the number of lower-level jobs. This, however, does not mean fewer jobs in the future. First of all, if improved productivity results in lower costs, it can also mean expanded levels of production. Secondly, new high-technology companies in such fields as electronics, communication, space, energy, etc., are creating many more new jobs, a high percentage of which are at technical and professional levels. So the trend from blue-collar to white-collar is likely to continue. The student, hearing or deaf, who does not prepare for these more challenging and rewarding jobs is more likely to fall victim to the advancing technology.

EDUCATION

Better education is clearly the key to preparing deaf students for a job market with a steadily increasing proportion of technical and professional positions. It is encouraging to see the wonderful developments at the college level. Not only has Gallaudet College continually added to and strengthened its educational offerings to keep pace with the demands of the labor market but, in the last twenty years, exciting new programs (e.g., the National Technical Institute for the Deaf [NTID], California State University at Northridge [CSUN], and a growing number of community colleges) have been inaugurated.

It is unfortunate that not enough hearing-impaired students make it to college. Clearly, a college education is not for everyone, hearing or deaf, but currently only a fraction of those hearing-impaired students who have the potential for doing college-level work actually get that opportunity. Unfortunately, regardless of how much intelligence or potential a person may have, undereducation will likely lead to underemployment.

The key bottleneck to further education occurs not at the college level, but at secondary and elementary levels, and sometimes even earlier. Methods must be found to equip a greater proportion of hearing-impaired students with the skills and background needed for success in college. It may be appropriate to lower somewhat the requirements for college entrance, to reduce the number of units that a student takes per quarter/semester, and to increase the number of years required to secure the degree. But the quality of the finished product, the hearing-impaired graduate, must not be sacrificed if he or she is to be competitive in the job market.

ATTITUDES

One question that continually arises when discussing this issue is whether or not the employment opportunites will be there for the qualified hearing-impaired applicant. Obviously, a healthy, growing economy provides more job opportunities than one that is depressed. But, as relevant as the strength of our economy is, the attitudes of employers toward deaf applicants are equally important. When it comes to employing deaf people, there are four attitudes that prevail.

1. *Resistive*—"We don't want any deaf employees around here; they are more bother than they are worth; this is a business, not a social welfare agency."
2. *Permissive*—"If a deaf person applies, sure, we'll consider him; but he better be able to function independently and in

standard ways; we're not about to bend the organization around to fit his needs."
3. *Accommodative*—"For a qualified deaf person, we can restructure the job somewhat so she won't need to use the phone; in department meetings we'll ask someone to sit with her and take notes; and maybe some people in her group will learn fingerspelling and some signs."
4. *Facilitative*—"Let's institute some special programs to augment accommodative measures; let's not just wait for qualified applicants, let's seek them out or perhaps we could even help deaf students to become qualified."

In regard to attitudes, it is inappropriate to ask, What is the attitude of the XYZ Company? Companies don't have attitudes, people have attitudes. Executive statements by high-level management tend to be accommodative if not facilitative. But what really counts are the attitudes of key individuals in personnel departments and those at the first and second levels of line management. These attitudes can differ from individual to individual within the same company as well as from department to department within the same company. Fortunately, over the past several years, there has been a steady shifting away from resistive and permissive attitudes toward the accommodative and facilitative, a trend that should continue in the years ahead.

EMPLOYMENT

Legislation designed to benefit handicapped persons has been on the books for a long time. Over the years, new state and federal provisions have been added to further correct various inequities. No law has done more to promote the cause of handicapped individuals than the Rehabilitation Act of 1973. This law and its subsequent amendments provide for increased rehabilitation services; the law also requires employers to take affirmative action on behalf of people with disabilities. "Hire the handicapped" is now more than a slogan—it is a directive. Handicapped people have become a minority whose job rights are written into the law of the land.

It would be regrettable, however, if progress could only come from adversarial relationships based on legal rights. Nevertheless, this legislation helps to set priorities for companies whose good intentions sometimes get deferred or sidetracked by the many other worthwhile activities that compete for attention.

John McLean, former professor at the Harvard Graduate School of Business Administration and chief executive officer of Continental Oil, once said that the primary purpose of business is to earn a profit—with decency. This means much more than avoiding the illegal or unethical; it means contributing positively to the general welfare. So, in addition to traditional business concerns about resource availability, production costs, and market acceptance, businesses must also consider the relatively new factors associated with environmental protection, consumer protection, and equality in employment.

The generally improving awareness of what hearing-impaired people can do in a variety of occupations, coupled with legislative promptings, is motivating business, industry, and government to seek out and hire qualified hearing-impaired applicants. The key word here is *qualified*. Clearly, applicants should not be hired simply because they cannot hear. But neither should they be given less consideration.

Deaf job seekers must be competitive with other available applicants in terms of their qualifications for the positions for which they apply. Technical and professional positions typically have educational prerequisites. To the extent that these are valid, they should not be waived or relaxed for deaf applicants.

INTERNSHIPS

One of the best ways for hearing-impaired students to strengthen their competitive position for permanent employment following graduation is by obtaining relevant work experience while they are still in college. This can sometimes be arranged through the placement office on campus. Both Gallaudet College and the National Technical Institute for the Deaf are particularly well equipped to assist their students in securing employment relevant to their academic majors. Gallaudet College has a special office called Experiential Programs Off Campus

(EPOC) specifically for this purpose. The National Technical Institute for the Deaf operates a National Center on Employment of the Deaf (NCED), a significant component of which is also devoted to this objective. This work experience is sometimes referred to as an internship or as cooperative education.

Since 1974, International Business Machines (IBM) has been actively involved with Gallaudet and NTID and, to a lesser extent, with other colleges around the country in a summer work-experience program for deaf college students. Those who are preparing for professional careers in computing, accounting, engineering, chemistry, and similar fields are given summer employment related to their course work. This is not a training program; students are expected to have completed enough relevant course work to be able, with some supervision, to function productively in the departments to which they are assigned.

In addition to using the knowledge and skills learned at college, the students involved in the IBM program develop greater technical competence as well as practical knowledge of the work environment. IBM, on the other hand, benefits from the work done by these summer employees and, in the process, becomes increasingly aware of the capabilities of deaf persons.

Each year, students work at more than 20 different IBM locations across the country. Thus, each year of the program, more and more IBM employees have the opportunity to become acquainted with a deaf co-worker and see first-hand that deafness has no impact on the ability of a qualified individual to function effectively in technical and professional assignments.

As these students are graduated from college, they have practical, relevant work experience to augment their academic credentials. They are thus better prepared for full-time regular employment and are much more likely to overcome the natural reservations of many potential employers.

ACCOMMODATION

Too frequently, the term *employing* is confused with *hiring*. Despite its critical importance, hiring someone is but a one-time activity in an ongoing process. Employing encompasses recruiting, evaluating, promoting, and, sometimes, firing. Employment is an interactive system whose various components may require special tuning in order to optimize the relationship between the employer and each individual employee. Although this is generally true for all, it is especially so for those who have disabilities.

Interpersonal communication on a one-to-one basis between a deaf person and a hearing manager or co-worker is rarely a problem at professional levels. The mode of communication may be different and perhaps a little slower than between two hearing people, but conversations take place with ease and clarity. Group meetings, however, are typically difficult for a deaf person in a hearing environment. Improvement in this area is occurring as more employers recognize the benefits of providing interpreter services for such occasions. The deaf employee is then better able to learn from what is being said in the meeting and is also able to contribute personal perspectives and expertise to the discussion.

The inability of a deaf person to use the telephone has frequently been used as justification for denying employment in certain job classifications. In many, if not in most, of these cases, a little imagination could have resolved the problem without compromising job expectations. A slight modification of the job description, or the installation of special telephone equipment or services, can usually result in job performance comparable to that of anyone else in the same or a similar position.

Students who obtain their academic degrees and enter the work force in technical and professional positions are typically well versed in the general aspects of their chosen fields. However, each company or government agency has its own way of using the standards and procedures that apply to the particular field. These practices must be learned on the job. On-the-job training is a continuing process that will be even more critical in the years ahead. Many technical and professional positions will be radically changed, some will even be eliminated, while new career opportunities will evolve.

One way for professionals, hearing or deaf, to stay abreast of new developments in their chosen fields is by reading the current technical or professional literature associated with their careers. In addition, many employers give their employees the opportunity to attend classes and seminars on new procedures, systems, technologies, products, or applications. The provision of interpreter services for such classes is becoming increasingly common.

Despite the training opportunities that many employees have, a great deal of what is learned on the job is learned informally by way of casual comments, hallway scuttlebutt, or lunchtime conversations. In the area of informal learning, the deaf person is likely to be at some disadvantage. As important as these informal channels of communication are to technical vitality, they are even more important for managerial awareness.

One of the opportunities open to deaf people entering the professional ranks is upward mobility. But, upward mobility does not necessarily imply management responsibility. In many organizations and career paths, there is a dual ladder by which one can receive promotions—a managerial ladder and a technical ladder. It is certainly not uncommon for a competent professional to be at a higher level and earn a higher salary than his or her manager.

PATERNALISM

There are a number of things that an employer can do to accommodate and facilitate the employment of deaf persons. But it would be inappropriate to imply that the deaf person does not have a corresponding responsibility to the employer. Unfortunately, in some instances, certain tendencies on the part of both the employee and employer can contribute to an unhealthy relationship (i.e., paternalism).

Some parents of children with disabilities, out of a sense of guilt or pity, or in simply trying to ease the way, overprotect their children and adopt expectations that are well below the children's capabilities. Teachers and advisors who are guilty of these same tactics reinforce and perpetuate a debilitating attitude of dependence among students, which can set the students up to fail to become qualified for the levels of employment that they could otherwise reach. Effective educators and rehabilitation counselors who work with handicapped persons encourage the development of independence in their students and clients.

Complete independence, however, is not only unrealistic, it is undesirable. Interdependence is better than independence. The degree to which one person is dependent on another varies from situation to situation, from job to job, and from person to person. If people are interdependent, they will sometimes be dependent on others, and others will sometimes be dependent on them. Being able to "hold up one's end" gives one pride in what is done and nurtures a sense of self-worth. This holds true whether or not a person has disabilities. Employers who expect less of deaf employees than they are capable of giving cheat the employees; and employers who accept less cheat themselves.

Summary

Major advances have been made during the past 20 years in the educational alternatives available to hearing-impaired students seeking higher education. Employers generally are more aware of deafness and more accepting of hearing-impaired applicants. Many are willing to make appropriate accommodations and some have instituted facilitative programs. Hearing-impaired persons in greater and greater numbers are preparing for and entering technical and professional careers in business, industry, and government.

Considerable progress has been made, but there is clearly much more to be done. Schools, agencies, and corporations cannot do it alone; it requires the enlightened and cooperative efforts of all, including hearing-impaired people themselves and the organizations that serve and represent them. Plans that are formulated and programs that are developed are apt to miss the mark if they are done *for* rather than *with* hearing-impaired workers. Working together, real progress can be made for all.

Chapter Nine
SUMMARY AND CONCLUSIONS

The results of the 1982 survey of hearing-impaired professional workers reveal that the respondents have achieved true professional status. A majority of them show all the significant indicators: parental socioeconomic status (and related expectations and privileges), high educational attainment, job classification, better than average salaries (though not as large as their hearing peers), and professional and community involvement. The major findings of the survey can be summarized as follows:

1. **Communication**
   a. A large majority (76.8%) of the respondents were employed in the deaf sector, where sign language is an accepted communication mode. These respondents reported having minimal communication difficulties.
   b. Almost 50% of the respondents who worked in an environment that required oral communication more than half of the time had good expressive and receptive speech skills.
   c. Respondents with a later age at onset of hearing loss usually had very intelligible speech but did not have good speech-reading skills.

2. **Education**
   a. The respondents were more highly educated than managerial and professional peers in the general population. This comparison was not made between homogeneous populations, however. The data used for hearing professional and managerial workers covered ages 16 years and older, whereas the hearing-impaired respondents were predominantly over 25 years of age.
   b. More than half of the hearing-impaired respondents had master's degrees. One probable reason for this is the licensing requirements for teachers of the hearing impaired. Ninety-two of the respondents held earned doctorates, not a large proportion compared to the general professional/managerial population, but a much larger number than existed among hearing-impaired people in 1960.

3. **Job Finding Techniques**
   a. As with their hearing peers, the largest proportion of the hearing-impaired respondents found their jobs through personal contacts.
   b. A larger percentage of the hearing-impaired respondents (27.2%) sought jobs through formal means than did hearing professionals (19%). When the respondents were divided into sectors, the proportion of those working in the deaf sector who sought jobs through formal means was identical to that of hearing persons (18.8%); the percentage of hearing sector respondents who used formal means was 34.1%.

4. **Job Sectors**
   a. More than 75% of the respondents worked in the deaf sector.
   b. A large percentage of the women respondents (87%) worked in the deaf sector.
   c. Of the respondents working in the deaf sector, 80.5% were teachers.
   d. Overall job satisfaction in each of the two sectors was about the same—respondents liked their jobs fairly well.

SUMMARY AND CONCLUSIONS 179

e. The amount of satisfaction gained by working in people-oriented jobs appeared to be greater in the deaf sector.
f. Respondents in the hearing sector were more satisfied with promotion and salary.
g. Respondents in the hearing sector earned a median salary $5,594 higher than those in the deaf sector.

5. **Occupational Mobility**
   a. A majority of the respondents were upwardly mobile occupationally. The greatest amount of upward mobility was gained by respondents from lower-class homes; conversely, the most downward mobility was experienced by respondents from upper-class homes.
   b. A multiple regression analysis indicated that five factors were statistically significant predictors of the respondents' educational attainment: age at onset of hearing impairment, extent of impairment, speech skill, college attended at baccalaureate level, and age. These factors can be termed intermediate links in the chain of relationships leading to occupational accomplishment.
   c. The strongest of the direct influences on respondents' occupational status was educational attainment. Father's occupation and respondents' gender also were early and direct influences.
   d. Postlingual deafness and less than severe hearing impairment tended to result in better speech skills. Respondents with good speech skills tended to choose a general rather than a specialized college for baccalaureate study. Graduates from general colleges more frequently earned graduate degrees; these, in turn, resulted in higher status jobs and higher salaries.

6. **Comparison Between Study Groups**
   a. The responses obtained from the 1960 and 1982 respondents who worked in the hearing sector were compared. All of the respondents compared were severely or profoundly deaf. About 81% of the 337 respondents in the 1982 group were college graduates; about 70% of the 87 respondents in the 1960 group were college graduates.

b. Median salaries (in 1982 dollars) were $26,291 in 1982 and $24,650 in 1960.
c. Median salaries in 1982 increased as each level of education increased; in 1960, graduate degrees brought higher earnings but no medians were available.
d. In the main, both groups reported high satisfaction with their jobs; they perceived little discrimination.
e. Sources other than this survey show a threefold increase in the numbers but not in the percentages of deaf people employed as part of the professional educational staff in schools and classes for deaf people. There appear to be more hearing-impaired educators in administrative, clinical, and other support activities in 1982 than there were in 1960.
f. Improved opportunities in higher education and active job placement efforts have increased industry awareness of the capabilities of deaf workers. More employers are willing to institute accommodative or facilitative programs to improve the productivity of deaf employees.

IMPLICATIONS OF THE FINDINGS

Drawing conclusions from the data presented in this book requires a few caveats. The group is not a scientifically selected sample since no corresponding benchmark data exists. Nor was it possible to conduct an exhaustive census. Yet, the large number of respondents and the high response rate, among the highest for national mail surveys of deaf adults (Schroedel, 1982a), give a certain validity to the careful generalizations extracted from these data. One more caveat—this discussion represents the opinions of the principal author only. Readers are entitled to disagree, but familiarity with the data analyzed and a lifetime of observation give some legitimacy to these thoughts.

In general, it is very encouraging to see the increase in the number of professional, technical, and managerial workers in the deaf community. These people are perfect examples of the benefits gained from more assertive attitudes among people with hearing impairments, expansion of collegiate options for higher education, scholarship funds, placement efforts, and mandatory employment laws that came about in the 1960s and 1970s.

The educational attainments of the 1982 respondents are high, remarkably so, and the statistics bode well for the future. The 92 doctorates in the 1982 group are a great improvement over the 5 in 1960, and the numerous master's degrees from various colleges and universities should help to obliterate the unthinking rejection of hearing-impaired students by many institutions of higher education.

The increasing number of deaf professionals in a wide variety of occupations can result in greater awareness and acceptance of hearing-impaired workers in higher level jobs, especially in the hearing sector. Jamison pointed out (in chap. 8) that the number of accommodative and facilitative employers has increased. Hearing-impaired workers can, by demonstrating competence and good working habits, widen this area of acceptance.

The implications are mixed for the deaf sector. Greater numbers of deaf people are employed in administrative positions (e.g., as superintendents of residential schools, coordinators of special programs in community colleges, and college vice presidents and deans). In time, we shall probably see a university provost or president. New service careers have opened, notably in social work. Careers in theatre were impractical and unthinkable in 1960, yet the National Theatre of the Deaf and individual deaf actors have won awards for excellence in recent years. This expansion of professional accomplishments has resulted from the hard work of individuals who have dared to aspire to develop in new directions.

In spite of the inroads made by deaf professionals, one group faces a doubtful future—the hearing-impaired teachers working in the deaf sector. Of the respondents employed in the deaf sector, 80.5% work in educational institutions. The number of hearing-impaired teachers has increased, but their proportion to the entire educational staff has decreased. An additional problem has developed in recent years—of all students in schools for the hearing impaired, the proportion attending residential schools has declined from 39.6% in 1975 (when PL 94-142 was enacted) to 30.9% in 1985 (Craig & Craig, 1976, 1986). This obviously shrinking market and the push by some federal officials for mainstreaming all handicapped pupils create a dark cloud on this particular horizon.

Deaf teachers have demonstrated their professional competence over the years, yet they are still faced with uninformed people who "know what is best" for them. Active political alliance with frustrated parents is one way to alleviate this discriminatory situation.

Demonstrated intergenerational upward mobility and the strength of education as a determinant of professional status imply that most qualified deaf persons can achieve high occupational status given the necessary determination. Future research on the nuts and bolts of mobility within the firm (e.g., how to grow on the job, secure promotions, and overcome communication barriers) might prove beneficial.

Job finding data imply the existence of a network for job seekers in the deaf sector and the lack or ineffectiveness of such a network in the hearing sector. Future research might replicate the present study and also examine the nature and extent of the networks. An obvious relationship exists between this sort of study and those related to occupational stereotyping by hearing-impaired youths. Findings in both areas imply a need for schools to invite professional and managerial workers from the hearing sector to the schools to offer a diversity of role models to their students.

The small but significant increase in the proportion of workers in the hearing sector who use manual communication with co-workers and the development of professional interpreting and telecommunication devices point to a reduction of barriers to employment in the hearing sector. Further aid might come in the improvement of computer networks and computers that are activated by speech.

The two decades preceding this study have constituted an era of humanitarian concern for minorities. Hearing-impaired people have benefited from this concern. The respondents examined in this text have met the challenge of the new opportunities offered them. Public awareness and defense of civil rights, though, are continuing needs. The price of occupational opportunities, like the price of liberty, is eternal vigilance by all concerned—researchers, educators, placement officials, and, most importantly, hearing-impaired workers themselves.

Appendix A
THE PROBLEM AND THE APPROACH

The two decades between 1960 and 1980 were a period of great advances and wider opportunities for people with hearing impairments in the United States. In relation to these conditions, certain questions arise: Were the results of this improved climate proportionate to the costs? Did hearing-impaired people rise to this improved environment and seize upon their opportunities? One way of looking into these questions is to examine the growth of employment successes (i.e., the increase of professional employment of hearing-impaired workers).

A study was conducted in 1982 to trace the growth of the population of deaf professional workers between 1960 and 1982 and to contrast the status of these workers. Certain characteristics of the 1982 group of respondents were compared to those of a 1960 group of 87 profoundly deaf individuals who worked in offices and laboratories where speech was the normal mode of communication.

The 1982 survey did not replicate the 1960 study. Time and monetary constraints made it necessary to undertake a mail survey rather than the lengthy interview method used in 1960. In addition, the criteria for inclusion went beyond profound deafness to include all hearing impairments. However, when making comparisons between the 1960 and 1982 groups, only those 1982 respondents who met the criteria used in 1960 were included.

ASSUMPTIONS

The basic assumption underlying the present study was that the number and variety of deaf professional workers had increased as educational and employment opportunities had broadened and as deaf sophistication and political assertiveness had grown. The components of the basic assumption were as follows:

1. The number of hearing-impaired persons professionally employed had increased over the number so employed in 1960.
2. The variety of professional positions filled by hearing-impaired workers was wider than in 1960.
3. Although hearing-impaired teachers worked mainly in residential schools for the deaf (as was the case in 1960), an increasing number of such teachers worked in day schools and classes (the public school system).
4. Educational attainment, as measured by academic degrees earned, was much higher than in 1960, although perhaps not as high as for the general population.
5. Hearing-impaired people had devoted more study to specific preparation for professional careers than they had in 1960.
6. Job seeking assistance was more available than it was in 1960.
7. Socioeconomic mobility was greater for hearing-impaired persons than for the general professional population.
8. Economic return (i.e., salaries and other monetary compensations) to hearing-impaired professionals was less than that received by the general professional population.
9. Most hearing-impaired professionals were well satisfied with their jobs.
10. Most of the hearing-impaired professionals working in an oral environment had very good oral communication skills.
11. A majority of hearing-impaired professional workers were in occupations serving hearing-impaired people.
12. Hearing-impaired professionals working in the deaf sector (i.e., serving people with hearing impairments) received less monetary compensation than those working in the hearing sector.
13. Job satisfaction among workers in the deaf sector was greater than that in the hearing sector.

METHOD

In 1960, a canvass was made of knowledgeable persons to secure names and addresses of hearing-impaired people who were thought to be in professional jobs. Potential respondents received a one-page questionnaire to determine such criteria as extent of deafness, job title and duties, and willingness to participate. Jobs were compared to the Census Bureau listing of "professional, technical and kindred workers" and "managers and administrators except farm." Those respondents whose jobs did not fit into these categories were dropped from the survey. The interviewers then visited the selected respondents, gave them the main questionnaire, and gave one to a co-worker who could hear.

The procedures used in 1982 involved a similar canvass to discover potential respondents. No preliminary questionnaire was used; the job titles and duties used to determine professional status were included in a single questionnaire. Since the new procedure brought in completed questionnaires from a great number of hearing-impaired professionals, it was decided to include respondents with all levels of impairment from all areas of employment. This meant, for example, inclusion of teachers of deaf children, social service workers, and ministers to hearing-impaired congregations. The mail survey technique also meant the exclusion of the assessments and remarks of colleagues, which were a worthy part of the 1960 study. In place of these, Mr. Steven L. Jamison, coordinator of the deaf program of International Business Machines Corporation, was asked to contribute a chapter about perspectives on employment of deaf people.

The names and addresses of possible respondents were secured from a number of sources. The following national lists and membership rosters provided most of the names.
1. Gallaudet College Alumni Survey, 1981.
2. National Technical Institute for the Deaf at Rochester Institute for Technology Alumni Feedback Survey. (Direct access to the NTID/RIT list was not possible because of confidentiality regulations. However, the NTID Planning and Evaluation Systems Office cooperated by mailing questionnaires to professional workers on their Alumni Feedback list.)

3. California State University, Northridge, listing of hearing-impaired professionals in industry and business.
4. Southwest Collegiate Institute for the Deaf faculty/staff roster and list of other known professionals.
5. Resource Directory of Handicapped Scientists (American Association for the Advancement of Science).
6. Educators with Disabilities (Merchant and Coriell).
7. National Listing of Disabled Artists, Educators, Administrators, and Advisors (National Committee—Arts for the Handicapped).
8. American Professional Society of the Deaf membership list.
9. Oral Deaf Adults Section, A. G. Bell Association for the Deaf, roster.
10. American Society of Deaf Social Workers roster.
11. Deaf Players Guide, National Theatre of the Deaf.

In addition to these organizations, mailing list information came from 14 state commissions or councils on deafness, 10 rehabilitation specialists for deaf clients, 10 national offices of religious programs, and 31 community leaders and others knowledgeable about deafness. All respondents were asked to name friends who held professional jobs; many did so. Considerable help in finding canvass sources came from the April 1982 Reference Issue of the *American Annals of the Deaf*.

All the names were entered on a computer mailing list. The program included a Soundex device to detect duplication of names. This device proved to be of special importance because individuals were often named on more than one list.

Hearing-impaired professionals in schools for the deaf were reached in a somewhat different manner. Schools were asked whether there were hearing-impaired professionals on their staffs. For those schools that did have such staff people, a bundle of questionnaires was sent to the administrative office for distribution to the proper persons there. The response from this group was very good: 288 administrators of educational institutions were sent questionnaires for distribution to an estimated 1,209 hearing-impaired professionals. This data came from the *American Annals of the Deaf*. Another listing of schools with hearing-impaired teachers was secured from the authors of *Teachers of the Deaf: Descriptive Profiles* (Corbett & Jensema, 1981). Both of these sources were coordinated with the mailing list of the Center for Assessment and Demographic Studies, Gallaudet College.

The mailing list was maintained through the Computer Center at Gallaudet College. The Gallaudet College Alumni Survey, 1981 (Armstrong, 1983), provided the basis for the mailing list. Names were added as they were received from the sources described above. A separate manual file of names was also maintained, using the identifying slips removed from the questionnaires after a code number had been assigned to each. The questionnaires were processed without names to preserve confidentiality.

In a pilot study, 50 questionnaires were sent to a randomly selected group; 44 responded. The questionnaire was then modified based on their sugggestions. The first mailing to schools for the deaf went out in November 1982. Other mailings were held back until this group could be recorded on the mailing list because considerable duplication was anticipated among teachers. The first mass mailing to individuals (2,654 questionnaires) was sent in mid-February 1983. On March 15, a second wave was mailed to those who had not yet responded.

Planning and Evaluation System officials at NTID/RIT sent 300 questionnaires to their alumni, followed by a second mailing. More questionnaires were sent out intermittently as names of potential respondents were received from the original survey respondents. This process continued until the cutoff date, October 31, 1983.

At the cutoff date, 3,247 valid records had been made, of which 134 had been returned as undeliverable. Several different groups of respondents (a total of 628) were eliminated as ineligible; these included nonprofessionals, retirees, part-time workers, unemployed persons, and persons who were not hearing impaired. From an eligible research population of 2,619, we found 1,735 respondents for the study, a response rate of 66.25%.

THE QUESTIONNAIRE

The questionnaire was kept relatively short and simple to encourage respondents to answer all the items. The aim was to develop a product that would take about half an hour to complete. Except for description of job duties, most questions were highly structured, permitting check marks for answers. The questionnaire is reprinted in Appendix C.

It is important to know the meaning of the terms used on the questionnaire. Some of these terms have different meanings, depending on the context in which they appear. For the purposes of this study, the terms can be defined as follows.

1. **Hearing impaired**—A generic term describing any significant hearing loss. Extent of impairment can be described by three terms. The relationship between these descriptions of hearing impairment and decibel measures is admittedly imperfect. A full description of how they are related for this study appears in Appendix B.

    a. *less than severe*—applies to those individuals whose hearing loss is moderate (i.e., less than 70 dB). They may have difficulty understanding a whisper in a quiet room or even loud speech into the better ear, but they can distinguish the sound of speech from other sounds without using a hearing aid.

    b. *severe*—applies to those individuals who have a hearing loss between 71–90 db. Without an aid, people with severe impairment may be able to tell one kind of noise from another, but they cannot distinguish speech.

    c. *profound*—applies to those individuals who have a hearing loss greater than 90 db. People with profound impairment lack usable hearing in ordinary, day-to-day communication without a hearing aid.

2. **Professional occupation**—An occupation included in the Census Bureau's 1970 occupational classification of "professional, technical, and kindred workers" and "managers and administrators, except farm." The 1980 Census classification was arranged and titled somewhat differently, but most of the job titles are the same as they were in 1970.

3. **Deaf community**—Schroedel (1984) has described the deaf community "as a configuration of overlapping social circles:

(1) with deaf persons socially active in the formal social, civic, and religious organizations which form the core of this community; (2) with deaf members less active in the formal organizations, but with either deaf spouses and or social networks of deaf friends who are loosely connected to the core; and (3) with isolated, transient, or non-signing oral deaf persons occupying the fringes of these formal and informal groupings. Local deaf communities are not only located in major towns and cities, but also have nationwide interconnections through national organizations, periodicals, special telephone networks, and postsecondary programs which attract deaf students from across the country. The national deaf community is the total of all deaf persons found in local communities."

4. **Deaf sector**—The part of the labor market that employs those respondents who either serve deaf people or work in situations where their deafness is applicable to their occupation (e.g., actors whose mime and body language is relevant to their job).

5. **Hearing sector**—The part of the labor market that employs respondents who work in corporations, government agencies, or self-owned businesses that serve the general public.

6. **Job finding methods**—The methods by which a worker first finds out about the job he or she currently holds.

7. **Personal contacts**—Information provided by a friend, acquaintance, or relative to a worker about a job opening.

8. **Direct application**—A job finding method in which the worker successfully applies directly to an employer without knowing if any specific job is available.

9. **Older workers**—Those workers over age 34.

10. **Younger workers**—Those workers under age 35.

ANALYSIS

Responses were coded by a simple numerical system, except for the occupational responses. Occupations were coded by the U.S. Census Bureau three-digit code for conversion into the Duncan Socioeconomic Scale and then by the 1980 code for comparisons with current Census data. Entries were made via a Demand-90 program for Gallaudet College's DEC-10 computer. Conversion to the 1022 program was made and data were analyzed using the Statistical Program for the Social Sciences.

Appendix B
DESCRIBING HEARING IMPAIRMENT

One aspect of hearing impairment that might affect a person's professional progress is the extent of the impairment. Those persons with less than severe impairment can communicate orally in many situations. With a hearing aid some may be able to converse about as well as a person with normal hearing. The severe and profound impairments are popularly described as deafness. A majority of deaf people depend on vision for their communication. Some are able to speechread and speak satisfactorily; others never master that art and use writing or sign language for communication.

Hearing impairment is most often measured on audiometers. The extent of hearing loss is measured in decibels (dB) for the better-ear average; the higher the decibel reading, the greater the loss. For a mail survey, audiograms are, of course, not practicable. Besides that, the respondents' perception of the usefulness of their hearing is an important measure in a socioeconomic study such as the present one. Therefore, we used the Hearing Ability Scale, devised by Schein, Gentile, and Haase (1970), to determine the respondents' extent of hearing impairment. The scale appeared on the questionnaire as follows:

6. Extent of deafness (Please answer each question either YES or NO by checking ONE choice per line. Answer the way you hear without a hearing aid.)
   a. Can you usually hear and understand what a person says without seeing his face if he whispers to you from across a quiet room? 1) ___ Yes 2) ___ No
   b. Can you usually hear and understand what a person says without seeing his face if he talks in a normal voice to you from across a quiet room? 1) ___ Yes 2) ___ No
   c. Can you usually hear and understand what a person says without seeing his face if he shouts to you from across a quiet room? 1) ___ Yes 2) ___ No
   d. Can you usually hear and understand a person if he speaks loudly into your better ear? 1) ___ Yes 2) ___ No
   e. Can you usually tell the sound of speech from other sounds and noises? 1) ___ Yes 2) ___ No
   f. Can you usually tell one kind of noise from another? 1) ___ Yes 2) ___ No
   g. Can you hear loud noises? 1) ___ Yes 2) ___ No

For purposes of analysis and narration it was necessary to have some brief verbal classification of extent of impairment. So, a conversion of scale scores to decibels and then to verbal description was attempted.

Schein, Gentile, and Haase (1970), in a study of 872 Gallaudet College students, compared the students' responses on the Hearing Ability Scale with their hearing loss (measured in decibels). Schein and Delk (1974) adapted the scale in developing a table of equivalences (see Table B-1).

In comparing the Hearing Ability Scale scores to audiometric decibel scores, Schein and Delk (1974) recognized that the elements measured by the two measuring devices were not the same.

> It is tempting to relate hearing levels for speech to each of the scale scores, but in doing so recognition must be given to the meaning of such correlation. The questions about hearing are a different means from audiometry of getting the same entity—functional hearing ability.

Hearing Scale II asks the individual to tell how he hears under particular circumstances. An audiological examination, on the other hand, presents him with pure tones at varying degrees of loudness . . . from which hearing for speech can be accurately, but not perfectly, predicted. Thus the Hearing Scale and the audiometer are both means of determining how well the individual can hear speech. They should be highly correlated, but at a level less than unity. For interpretation of the Hearing Scale scores, audiometric measures are helpful. Similarly, the Hearing Scale assists in explicating the functional meaning of a given hearing level for speech. (pp. 138–139)

In short, like apples and oranges, the two measures are not identical, but, like the fruit, they have similarities.

Karchmer, Milone, and Wolk (1974) devised the three categories of impairment used in the 1982 study—less than severe (less than 70 dB), severe (71–90 dB) and profound (more than 90 dB). Their classification and a rough equivalence in Hearing Ability Scale scores are shown in Table B-2.

Table B-1
Mean Better-Ear Average, in Decibels, and
Standard Deviations for Scores on Hearing Scale II

Scale Score[a]	Mean Better-Ear Average in Decibels, ISO	Standard Deviation
1	13.7	11.7
2	28.3	16.3
3	42.2	16.7
4	63.3	18.5
5–8	81.8	20.5

Note. From *The Deaf Population of the United States* (p. 139) by J. D. Schein and M. T. Delk, 1974, Silver Spring, MD: National Association of the Deaf. Copyright 1974 by NAD. Reprinted by permission.

[a]Score refers to the highest item in Hearing Scale II (Schein, Gentile, & Haase, 1970, p. 40) to which the person responds Yes . . . Thus a score of 1 is assigned if a person responds Yes to item 1 (a) (and, therefore, to all subsequent items). A score of 2 means that the respondent answered No to the first item (a) and Yes to all remaining items. A score of 8 is given when all seven answers to the scale are negative.

Table B-2
Hearing Ability Scale Scores Converted to
BEA Decibels and Extent of Impairment (in Words)

Hearing Ability Scale Score	Better-Ear Average in Decibels, ISO	Extent of Impairment
2–4	Less than 70 dB	Less than Severe
5 & 6	71–90 dB	Severe
7 & 8	More than 90 dB	Profound

A hearing loss of less than 27 decibels is considered to be within normal limits of hearing (Karchmer, Milone, & Wolk, 1974); therefore all respondents answering *yes* to question *a* in the Hearing Ability Scale were eliminated from the group. The scale scores 5–8 (Yes at lines *d, e, f, g*, or none at all) are divided arbitrarily into severe and profound, and the equivalences are not precise. For narrative purposes the three classes will be satisfactory. In some cases, respondents answered a few queries with a *no*, then checked a *yes*, then next a *no*. In such cases, the first *yes* was taken as the cutoff; subsequent *no* answers were disregarded.

For some people, hearing impairment is a condition into which they are born; for others sickness, especially high fevers, causes sudden, extensive loss of hearing; for still others, the onset of the disability is gradual. Hence, the questionnaire for this study asked:

How old were you when you began to have serious trouble hearing or became deaf?

1) ___ Less than 1 year old
2) ___ 1 and under 3 years old
3) ___ 3 and under 6 years old
4) ___ 6 and under 12 years old
5) ___ 12 and under 19 years old
6) ___ 19 years old or older

Persons whose impairment had occurred prior to age 19 were called *prevocationally deaf* by Schein and Delk (1974).

# Appendix C
PROFESSIONAL EMPLOYMENT QUESTIONNAIRE

Background Information

1. What year were you born? _____

2. What is your sex? (1) ____ Male (2) ____ Female

3. What is your race? (1) ____ White (2) ____ Black
   (3) ____ Hispanic (4) ____ Asian (5) ____ American Indian
   (6) ____ Other (Please explain) ____

4. a. What was the name of your father's usual occupation when you were about age 16? If he had more than one occupation, name the one which was the most important.
   _____

   b. What were the tasks which he did on this job most of the time?
   _____

   c. What was the name of your mother's occupation when you were about age 16?
   _____

   d. What tasks did she perform?
   _____

Hearing

5. How old were you when you began to have serious trouble hearing or became deaf?

   (1) ____ Less than 1 year old
   (2) ____ 1 and under 3 years old
   (3) ____ 3 and under 6 years old
   (4) ____ 6 and under 12 years old
   (5) ____ 12 and under 19 years old
   (6) ____ 19 years old or older

6. Extent of deafness (Please answer each question either YES or NO by checking ONE choice per line. Answer the way you hear without a hearing aid.)

   a. Can you usually hear and understand what a person says without seeing his face if he whispers to you from across a quiet room?   (1) ____ Yes   (2) ____ No

   b. Can you usually hear and understand what a person says without seeing his face if he talks in a normal voice to you from across a quiet room?   (1) ____ Yes   (2) ____ No

   c. Can you usually hear and understand what a person says without seeing his face if he shouts to you from across a quiet room?   (1) ____ Yes   (2) ____ No

   d. Can you usually hear and understand a person if he speaks loudly into your better ear?   (1) ____ Yes   (2) ____ No

   e. Can you usually tell the sound of speech from other sounds and noises?   (1) ____ Yes   (2) ____ No

   f. Can you usually tell one kind of noise from another?
      (1) ____ Yes   (2) ____ No

   g. Can you hear loud noises?   (1) ____ Yes   (2) ____ No

Communication

7. What percent of your daily communication during working hours is with persons who do not use sign language?

   (1) ____ 0–24%   (2) ____ 25–49%   (3) ____ 50–74%
   (4) ____ 75–100%

8. What percent of your social contacts away from work are with people who do not use sign language?

   (1) ____ 0–24%   (2) ____ 25–49%   (3) ____ 50–74%
   (4) ____ 75–100%

9. When you want to communicate *to hearing co-workers*, which method below do you use the most?

   Please check one method

Writing	____
Talking	____
Sign language without speech	____
Sign language with speech at the same time	____
Fingerspelling only	____
Other (Please describe) _____	____

10. When hearing co-workers communicate to you, which method do they use most often?

    Please check one method

Writing	____
Talking	____
Sign language without speech	____
Sign language with speech at the same time	____
Fingerspelling only	____
Other (Please describe) _____	____

11. Which one of the sentences below best describes how well you understand the speech of hearing co-workers most of the time, during one-to-one conversations? (Check one)

   (1) ____ I understand almost everything they say, no matter how they say it.
   (2) ____ I understand a short conversation, when it is spoken carefully.
   (3) ____ I understand only a short, simple sentence spoken very carefully.
   (4) ____ I understand only a word or two now and then.

12. Which one of the sentences below best describes how well your hearing co-workers seem to understand your speech in your usual working environment? (Check one)

   (1) ____ They don't have to listen carefully to understand most everything I say.
   (2) ____ They understand almost everything I say but often ask me to repeat.
   (3) ____ They understand only a word or two now and then.
   (4) ____ None of these (Please describe) _____

13. From whom did you *first* learn to sign? (Please check one)

   (1) ____ Family (parents or siblings)
   (2) ____ Friends outside of school
   (3) ____ School staff or teacher
   (4) ____ School pupils
   (5) ____ At college
   (6) ____ Other (whom?)
   (7) ____ I do not sign

Education

14. Which of the following best describes the type of school from which you received your high school diploma? (Check one)

   (1) ____ Residential high school for deaf students only
   (2) ____ Day high school with program for deaf students only
   (3) ____ General high school with program for deaf students as well as hearing

(4) ____ General high school without a program for deaf students
(5) ____ General boarding school or preparatory academy
(6) ____ Other (Please describe) _____

15. Circle below the number which shows the highest level of education (by grade or year as usually measured) which you have completed. (Circle one)

                                              College
Elementary and high school Undergraduate MA/MS JD etc. Doctorate
1 2 3 4 5 6 7 8 9 10 11 12   13 14 15 16   17 18   19   20 21

16. For each college degree or program which you have completed, please provide the following information:

	Major	Name of College	Year Completed
Certificate			
Associate Degree			
BA/BS			
Other			
MA/MS (1 year)			
MA/MS (2 years)			
Other			
Doctorate			

17. During your studies at college(s) other than Gallaudet or NTID, what special aids did you have? (Check all that apply)

(1) ____ Interpreters
(2) ____ Note takers
(3) ____ Tutors
(4) ____ Counselors
(5) ____ Favorable seating
(6) ____ Speech and hearing centers
(7) ____ Professors who knew something about deafness
(8) ____ Attendance at some classes not required
(9) ____ Extra copies of lecture notes
(10) ____ Other (What?) _____

Occupation

First Professional Job: Now some questions about the first full-time professional job on which you worked after you had completed your first college degree.

18. When did you start your first professional job as described above? (Year) _____

19. Who helped you the most in getting your first full-time professional job? (Check one).
    (1) ___ College placement officer
    (2) ___ Other college faculty or staff
    (3) ___ Rehabilitation counselor
    (4) ___ Employment office
    (5) ___ Family
    (6) ___ Friend
    (7) ___ Found the job myself
    (8) ___ Other (Specify)

20. What was the title of that first professional job?
    _____

21. What were the tasks or duties that you did on this job most of the time?
    _____

22. Which words below best describe your first employer? (Check one)
    (1) ___ Private business
    (2) ___ Self-employed (own business)
    (3) ___ Educational institution
    (4) ___ Government (federal, state, or local—non-educational)

23. How many hours a week do you work for pay now? (Check one)
    (1) ___ less than 35 hours   (2) ___ 35 hours or more

Job Now: If the job you have now is *different from your first job* as described in Questions 20–22, please now answer Questions 24, 25, 26, and 27.

PROFESSIONAL EMPLOYMENT QUESTIONNAIRE

If your job now is the *same one as your first job*, do not answer Questions 24–27. Go to Question 28.

24. What is the title of this job you have now?
    _____

25. What are the tasks or duties that you do on this job most of the time?
    _____

26. How many persons do you supervise? (Circle one)

    1 2 3 4 5 6 7 8 or more

27. Which words below best describe the employer you work for now? (Check one)

    (1) ____ Private business
    (2) ____ Self-employed (own business)
    (3) ____ Educational institution
    (4) ____ Government (federal, state, or local—non-educational)

28. In what year did you begin the job you have now?
    _____

29. Before taxes and other subtractions (social security, health insurance, charity donations, etc.) in 1982, how much was your salary, as shown on your W-2 form? (Check one group which indicates your salary).

    (1) ____ Under $10,000
    (2) ____ $10,000–14,999
    (3) ____ $15,000–19,999
    (4) ____ $20,000–24,999
    (5) ____ $25,000–29,999
    (6) ____ $30,000–34,999
    (7) ____ $35,000–39,999
    (8) ____ $40,000–44,999
    (9) ____ $45,000–49,999
    (10) ____ $50,000 and over

30. There are a number of aids to communication listed below. How do you rate these aids as used in your working environment? (Check one for each line).

	Do not have	Very helpful	Fairly helpful	Not helpful
Telephone with visual display (TDD/TTY)	___	___	___	___
Interpreter	___	___	___	___
Telephone amplifier	___	___	___	___
Hearing aid	___	___	___	___
Secretary (notes for conferences/phone)	___	___	___	___
Co-worker (notes for conferences/phone)	___	___	___	___
Agenda to read before meeting	___	___	___	___
Summary of meeting given you afterwards	___	___	___	___

Other (Please describe) _____

31. How many times have you been promoted to a new job at your present place of employment?
    _____

32. Have you received any merit raises or awards in the job you now have?
    (1) ___ Yes   (2) ___ No

33. How much do you like each of these situations? (Check one for each line)

	Like very much	Like a little	Dislike a little	Dislike very much	Does not apply
Chances for promotion	___	___	___	___	___
The kind of work you are doing	___	___	___	___	___
Your supervisors	___	___	___	___	___
Colleagues who work *with* you	___	___	___	___	___

People who work *for* you   ____ ____ ____ ____ ____
Your salary   ____ ____ ____ ____ ____

34. How often have you experienced unfair rejection by employers in each of the job activities listed below? (Check one for each line)

	Very often	Often	Sometimes	Almost never	Never
Hiring	____	____	____	____	____
Promotion	____	____	____	____	____
Training on the job	____	____	____	____	____
Work evaluation	____	____	____	____	____
Communication at work	____	____	____	____	____
Salary	____	____	____	____	____

Dream job: Many of us hope for a dream job. What are your hopes?

35. Write the job title that best describes your dream job.

_____

36. Describe some of the tasks which you would do most of the time if you were working on your dream job.

_____

Activities in Organizations

37. Write in below the names of professional associations or societies to which you paid dues in 1982. For each organization check all activities that you did. Please write out full names of organizations.

	Attended meetings	Served on committees	Was elected officer	None of these
_____	____	____	____	____
_____	____	____	____	____
_____	____	____	____	____
_____	____	____	____	____

38. Do the same for community organizations such as civic associations, service clubs, NAD, RID, state associations, and such.

	Attended meetings	Served on committees	Was elected officer	None of these
_____	____	____	____	____
_____	____	____	____	____
_____	____	____	____	____
_____	____	____	____	____

THANK YOU! If you wish, please write comments or further information below or on separate sheets.

Appendix D
DISTRIBUTION OF OCCUPATIONS— ALL RESPONDENTS

EXECUTIVE, ADMINISTRATIVE, AND MANAGERIAL OCCUPATIONS

Administrators and officials, public administration	7
Financial managers	2
Administrators, education and related fields	13
Managers, medicine and health	3
Managers and administrators, n.e.c. [not elsewhere classified]	34
*Directors, state offices for the deaf and departments in business firms	97
*Vice presidents and deans, college	14
*Coordinators, junior college programs	18

MANAGEMENT-RELATED FIELDS

Accountants and auditors	63
Other financial officers	6
Management analysts	2
Buyers, wholesale and retail trade except farm products	1

* indicates special categories to reflect special employment situations experienced by hearing-impaired professional workers.

Inspectors and compliance officers, except construction 5
*Supervising teachers, principals, coordinators of programs 77
*Coordinators of programs not in a school for the deaf 20
Management-related occupations, n.e.c. 3

PROFESSIONAL SPECIALTY OCCUPATIONS

Architects 7

Engineers, Surveyors, and Mapping Scientists
   Aerospace 3
   Metallurgical and materials 2
   Petroleum 1
   Civil 4
   Electrical and electronic 1
   Industrial 3
   Mechanical 1
   Engineers, n.e.c. 14

Mathematical and Computer Scientists
   Computer systems analysts and scientists 54
   Operations and systems researchers and analysts 8
   Statisticians 2
   Mathematical scientists 9

Natural Scientists
   Physicists and astronomers 1
   Chemists, except biochemists 15
   Geologists and geodesists 2
   Biological and life scientists 8
   Medical scientists 1

Health Diagnosing Occupations
   Physicians 3
   Dentists 4
   Veterinarians 1
   Health diagnosing practitioners, n.e.c. 3

Health Assessment and Treatment Occupations
   Registered nurses 1
   Therapists, n.e.c. 3

Teachers, Postsecondary
  Biological science teachers   2
  Chemistry teachers   5
  Physics teachers   2
  Psychology teachers   2
  Economics teachers   1
  Sociology teachers   2
  Social science teachers, n.e.c.   3
  Engineering teachers   2
  Mathematical science teachers   9
  Medical science teachers   1
  Health specialties teachers   1
  Business, commerce, and marketing teachers   5
  Art, drama, and music teachers   5
  Physical education teachers   1
  Education teachers   5
  English teachers   14
  Foreign language teachers   1
  Teachers, postsecondary, n.e.c.   14
  Teachers, postsecondary, subject not specified   22

Teachers, Except Postsecondary
  Teachers, prekindergarten and kindergarten   17
  Teachers, elementary school   154
  Teachers, secondary school   187
  Teachers, special education   1
  Teachers, n.e.c.   318

Counselors
  Educational and vocational   131

Librabrians, Archivists, and Curators
  Librarians   33
  Archivists and curators   3

Social Scientists and Urban Planners
  Psychologists   12
  Sociologists   1
  Social scientists, n.e.c.   11

Social, Recreation, and Religious Workers
	Social workers	27
	Recreation workers	8
	Clergy	22
	Religious workers	9

Lawyers and Judges
	Lawyers	8

Writers, Artists, Entertainers, and Athletes
	Authors	2
	Designers	23
	Actors and directors	10
	Painters, sculptors, crafts workers, and printmakers	2
	Photographers	4
	Artists, performers, and related workers, n.e.c.	11
	Editors and reporters	8
	Public relations specialists	10

TECHNICIANS AND RELATED SUPPORT OCCUPATIONS

Health Technologists and Technicians
	Clinical laboratory technologists and technicians	14
	Dental hygienists	1
	Health record technologists and technicians	2
	Health technologists and technicians, n.e.c.	11

Technologists and Technicians, Except Health
	Engineering technicians, n.e.c.	5
	Drafting occupations	16

Science Technicians
	Biological	1

Technicians, Except Health, Engineering, and Science
	Computer programmers	49
	Technicians, n.e.c.	11

TOTAL	1735

Appendix E
DISTRIBUTION OF OCCUPATIONS—1982 COMPARISON GROUP

EXECUTIVE, ADMINISTRATIVE, AND MANAGERIAL OCCUPATIONS

Administrators and officials, public administration	6
Financial managers	1
Administrators, education and related fields	2
Managers, medicine and health	2
Managers and administrators, n.e.c.	23

MANAGEMENT-RELATED FIELDS

Accountants and auditors	50
Other financial officers	4
Management analysts	1
Buyers, wholesale and retail trade except farm products	1
Inspectors and compliance officers, except construction	2
Management-related occupations, n.e.c.	2

PROFESSIONAL SPECIALTY OCCUPATIONS

Architects	5
Engineers, Surveyors, and Mapping Scientists	
Aerospace	3
Metallurgical and materials	2
Petroleum	1
Civil	3
Industrial	2
Mechanical	1
Engineers, n.e.c.	12
Mathematical and Computer Scientists	
Computer systems analysts and scientists	45
Operations and systems researchers and analysts	7
Statisticians	2
Mathematical scientists	8
Natural Scientists	
Chemists, except biochemists	15
Geologists and geodesists	1
Biological and life scientists	7
Medical scientists	1
Health Diagnosing Occupations	
Physicians	2
Dentists	3
Health Assessment and Treatment Occupations	
Registered nurses	1
Therapists, n.e.c.	3
Teachers, Postsecondary	
Medical science teachers	1

Teachers, Except Postsecondary
   Teachers, elementary school   1
   Teachers, n.e.c.   1

Counselors
   Educational and vocational   1

Librarians, Archivists, and Curators
   Librarians   8
   Archivists and curators   1

Social Scientists and Urban Planners
   Psychologists   1
   Social scientists, n.e.c.   1

Social, Recreation, and Religious Workers
   Recreation workers   1

Lawyers and Judges
   Lawyers   6

Writers, Artists, Entertainers, and Athletes
   Designers   2
   Painters, sculptors, crafts workers, and printmakers   2
   Photographers   2
   Artists, performers, and related workers, n.e.c.   2

TECHNICIANS AND RELATED SUPPORT OCCUPATIONS

Health Technologists and Technicians
   Clinical laboratory technologists and technicians   12
   Dental hygienists   1
   Health record technologists and technicians   2
   Health technologists and technicians, n.e.c.   8

Technologists and Technicians, Except Health
Engineering technicians, n.e.c. 5
Drafting occupations 13

Science Technicians
Biological 1

Technicians, Except Health, Engineering, and Science
Computer programmers 41
Technicians, n.e.c. 6

TOTAL 337

Appendix F
INDEXES OF JOB SATISFACTION AND REJECTION

Most of the tables in this book present the data in percentages rather than in absolute figures. In order to calculate indexes, however, absolute figures are necessary. This appendix demonstrates how indexes of job satisfaction and of rejection can be calculated. The tables in this appendix are similar to Tables 6 and 7, except for the use of figures instead of percentages.

To calculate the index of job satisfaction, the intensity of respondents' like or dislike for each factor is represented by weighting the levels as follows: Dislike very much, -2; dislike a little, -1; does not apply, 0; like a little, $+1$; like very much, $+2$. The algebraic sum of the weighted values is then divided by the absolute sum of the unweighted values. The resulting indexes will have a range of likes between -2 and $+2$; the negative values indicate dislike and the positive values indicate like (see Table F-1). A sample calculation would look as follows:

$$\frac{-2(84) - 1(85) + 0(577) + 1(269) + 2(650)}{84 + 85 + 269 + 650 + 577} = \frac{1316}{1665} = 0.79$$

Interpreting these indexes, it might be said that the respondents like their work, their colleagues, and supervisors quite well. Their subordinates do not rank as highly as other co-workers because the "does not apply" category reduces the index. Respondents are mildly pleased with salaries and promotions, the latter also being affected by the "does not apply" category. By summing the indexes and dividing by 6, an overall approximation of total job satisfaction can be found. In this case the overall index is 1.24.

An index of perceived rejection can also be made from the data collected from the respondents (see Table F-2). In this case, the range of weights is 0 to 4—0 = never and 4 = very often. Weighted figures are summed and then divided by the sum of the absolute figures.

The calculation for hiring was done as follows:

$$\frac{0(682) + 1(326) + 2(402) + 3(136) + 4(83)}{682 + 326 + 402 + 136 + 83} = \frac{1870}{1629} = 1.15$$

Table F-1
Job Satisfaction as Perceived by Respondents

Degree of Liking	Chance for Promotion	Kind of Work	Super-visors	Colleagues	Subor-dinates	Salary
Like very much	650	1369	1053	1250	844	717
Like a little	269	242	393	323	196	586
Dislike a little	85	74	113	40	27	230
Dislike very much	84	22	58	9	14	147
Does not apply	577	7	86	74	574	22
Total	1665	1714	1703	1696	1655	1702
Index of job satisfaction	0.79	1.67	1.33	1.63	1.11	0.88

Table F-2
Extent of Rejection Perceived by Respondents

Perceived Degree of Rejection	Hiring	Promotion	Training	Evaluation	Communication	Salary
Never	682	687	863	745	527	702
Almost never	326	319	325	410	368	355
Sometimes	402	361	275	335	510	390
Often	136	137	102	106	151	117
Very often	83	67	35	44	92	50
Total	1629	1571	1600	1640	1648	1614
Index of rejection	1.15	1.09	0.83	0.96	1.34	1.04

Reference List

Adler, E. P. (Ed.). (1969). Deafness: Research and professional training programs on deafness sponsored by the Department of Health, Education, and Welfare. *Journal of Rehabilitation of the Deaf Monograph 2*(5, Serial No. 1).

Advisory Committee on the Education of the Deaf. (1965). *Education of the deaf: A report to the Secretary of Health, Education, and Welfare*. Washington, DC: U.S. Department of Health, Education, and Welfare.

Albrecht, C. L., & Levy, J. A. (1984). A sociological perspective of physical disability. In J. L. Ruffini (Ed.), *Advances in medical social research* (Vol. 2). New York: Gordon & Branch.

Allen, R. E., & Keaveny, T. J. (1980). The relative effectiveness of alternative job sources. *Journal of Vocational Behavior, 16*, 18–32.

Alwin, D. F. (1974). College effects on educational and occupational attainments. *American Sociological Review, 39*(2), 210–223.

Armstrong, D. F. (1981). *1980–81 Gallaudet alumni survey: Introductory report* (Report No. 81-6). Washington, DC: Gallaudet College Planning Office.

Armstrong, D. F. (1983). Income and occupations of deaf former college students. *Journal of Rehabilitation of the Deaf, 17*(1), 8–15.

Barnartt, S. N. (1982). The socioeconomic status of deaf women. Are they doubly disadvantaged? In J. Christiansen & J. Egelston-Dodd (Eds.), *Socioeconomic status of the deaf population*. Washington, DC: Gallaudet College.

Barnartt, S. B., & Christiansen, J. B. (1985). The socioeconomic status of deaf workers: A minority group perspective. *Social Science Journal, 32*, 19–32.

Bell scholarship granted. (1968). *Volta Review, 70*, 82.

Blau, P. M., & Duncan, O. D. (1967). *The American occupational structure*. New York: Wiley.

Brown, D. G. (1965). *Academic labor markets*. Washington, DC: Department of Labor, Office of Manpower, Automation, and Training.

Brown, R. (1973). *A first language: The early stages*. Cambridge: Harvard University Press.

Bureau of the Census. (1971a). *Alphabetical index of industries and occupations: 1970 census of population*. Washington, DC: Government Printing Office.

Bureau of the Census. (1971b). *1970 census of the population, occupation classification*. [Leaflet]

Bureau of the Census (1980, June 10). *1980 Census of population: Occupational classification system, detailed occupational categories*. [Leaflet]

Bureau of the Census. (1981). *Statistical abstract of the United States* (102d edition). Washington, DC: Government Printing Office.

Bureau of Labor Statistics. (1980). *Occupational projections and training data* (Bulletin 2052). Washington, DC: Government Printing Office.

Bureau of Labor Statistics. (1983, January). *Educational attainment of workers, March 1982*. (Special Labor Force Report). Washington, DC: Department of Labor.

Bureau of Labor Statistics. (1984, May 22). *Consumer price index— Urban wage earners and clerical workers*. Washington, DC: Department of Labor.

Bureau of Labor Statistics. (n.d.). *Weekly earnings of employed wage and salary workers who usually work full-time by detailed (3-digit Census code) occupation (1982 annual averages).*
Califano, J. A. (1979, March 23). Statement. [News release]. Washington, DC: Department of Health, Education and Welfare.
Carr-Saunders, A. M. (1955). Metropolitan conditions and traditional professional relationships. In R. M. Fisher (Ed.), *The metropolis in modern life* (pp. 279–288). New York: Doubleday.
Chubon, R. A., & Black, B. L. (1985). A comparison of career awareness development in deaf residential school students and nondisabled public school students. *Journal of Rehabilitation of the Deaf, 18*(4), 1–5.
Cook, L., & Rossett, A. (1975). The sex role attitudes of deaf adolescent women and their implications for vocational choice. *American Annals of the Deaf, 120*, 341–345.
Cooley, C. H. (1964). The primary group. In L. A. Coser & B. Rosenberg (Eds.), *Sociological theory: A book of readings* (2nd ed.). New York: Macmillan.
Corbett, E. C., Jr., & Jensema, C. J. (1981). *Teachers of the deaf: Descriptive profiles.* Washington, DC: Gallaudet College Press.
Craig, H. B. (1983). Parent-infant education in schools for deaf children: Report of CEASD survey. *American Annals of the Deaf, 128*, 82–98.
Craig, W. H., & Craig, H. B. (Eds.). (1975). Tabular summary of schools and classes in the United States. *American Annals of the Deaf, 121*, 144.
Craig, W. H., & Craig, H. B. (Eds.). (1983). Tabular summary of schools and classes in the United States. *American Annals of the Deaf, 128*, 210–211.
Craig, W. H., & Craig, H. B. (Eds.). (1986). Tabular summary of schools and classes in the United States. *American Annals of the Deaf, 131*, 134–135.
Crammatte, A. B. (Ed.). (1965). *Guidelines for establishment of rehabilitation facilities for the deaf: A manual based on workshops at Fort Monroe, Virginia, and Delavan, Wisconsin, in 1959 and 1962.* Washington, DC: Vocational Rehabilitation Administration.
Crammatte, A. B. (1968). *Deaf persons in professional employment.* Springfield, IL: Charles C. Thomas.

Crammatte, A. B. (1978). Comments, questions and answers. *American Annals of the Deaf, 123*, 911.
Crammatte, A. B. (1979). Comments, questions and answers. *American Annals of the Deaf, 124*, 416.
Crammatte, A. B. (1980). Comments, questions and answers. *American Annals of the Deaf, 125*, 519.
Crammatte, A. B. (1982, May 15). Graduate fellowship fund committee. *Gallaudet Alumni Newsletter, 16*(14), 7–8.
Crammatte, A. B., & Schreiber, L. F. (1961). *Proceedings of the workshop on community development through organizations of and for the deaf.* Washington, DC: Gallaudet College.
Croneberg, C. G. (1976). The linguistic community. In W. C. Stokoe, D. C. Casterline, & C. G. Croneberg (Eds.), *A dictionary of American Sign Language on linguistic principles* (pp. 297–311). Silver Spring, MD: Linstok Press.
Davila, R., & Brill, R. G. (1976). Guest editorial. *American Annals of the Deaf, 121*, 361.
Deaf American. (1973, June). *25*(10).
Deaf man chosen to Office of Vocational Rehabilitation. (1945, September). *The Cavalier, 6*(9), 1. (Available from Merrill Learning Center, Gallaudet University, Washington, DC 20002; or National Center on Deafness, California State University, Northridge, CA 91330)
Degrell, R. E., & Ouellette, S. E. (1981). The role and function of a counselor in residential schools for the deaf. *American Annals of the Deaf, 126*, 64–68.
Department of Labor. (1977). *Dictionary of occupational titles* (4th ed.). Washington, DC: Government Printing Office.
DeSchweinetz, D. (1932). *How workers find jobs.* Philadelphia: University of Pennsylvania Press.
Di Lorenzo, L., & Welsh, W. (1981). *How long to receive a degree?* (Concept paper: Follow-up Report No. 1). Rochester, NY: NTID Institutional Planning and Research.
Doctor, P. V. (1961). Tabular summary of schools and classes in the United States. *American Annals of the Deaf, 106*, 163.
Duncan, O. D. (1961a). Properties and characteristics of the socioeconomic index. In A. J. Reiss (Ed.), *Occupations and social status* (pp. 109–138). New York: Free Press.

Duncan, O. D. (1961b). A socioeconomic index for all occupations. In A. J. Reiss, (Ed.), *Occupations and social status* (pp. 139–161). New York: Free Press.

Duncan, O. D., Featherman, D. L., & Duncan, B. (1972). *Socioeconomic background and achievement.* New York: Seminar Press.

Duprez, D. (1971). Occupational prestige and its correlates as conceived by deaf, female vocational students. *American Annals of the Deaf, 116,* 408–412.

Egelston-Dodd, J. (1974). *A comparison of occupational sex role stereotypes for deaf and hearing junior high school students.* Paper presented at the annual meeting of the New York State Association for the Education of the Deaf, New York City.

Egelston-Dodd, J. (1977a). Overcoming occupational stereotypes related to sex and deafness. *American Annals of the Deaf, 122,* 489–491.

Egelston-Dodd, J. (1977b). A philosophy and paradigm for a career education program for deaf learners. *Journal of Career Education, III*(4), 34–40.

Egelston-Dodd, J. (1978). *An intervention program for occupational stereotyping by deaf students.* Paper presented at National Science Foundation Working Conference on Science in Education for Handicapped Students, Washington, DC.

Falberg, R. N. (Ed.). (1967). Developments and programs. *Journal of Rehabilitation of the Deaf, 1*(1), 64.

Featherman, D. L., & Hauser, E. M. (1975). *Opportunity and change.* New York: Academic Press.

Frisina, R. D. (1971). Introduction to the National Technical Institute for the Deaf. *Journal of Rehabilitation of the Deaf, 4*(3), 154–160.

Gallagher, B. G. (1949). *The federal government and higher education of the deaf: A progress report on Columbia Institution for the Deaf, with proposals for action to complete the study.* Washington, DC: [s.n.].

Gallaudet College. (1976). *Gallaudet College self-evaluation report.* Washington, DC: Author.

Gallaudet College. (1980). *The Gallaudet College self-evaluation report for the 1981 re-accreditation review: A report to the Post-*

Secondary Commission of the Middle Atlantic Association of Colleges and Schools. Washington, DC: Author.
Gannon, J. R. (1981). *Deaf heritage: A narrative history of deaf America.* Silver Spring, MD: National Association of the Deaf.
Granovetter, M. S. (1973). The strength of weak ties. *American Journal of Sociology, 8,* 1360–1380.
Granovetter, M. S. (1974). *Getting a job: A study of contacts and careers.* Cambridge: Harvard University Press.
Griffin, L. J., & Alexander, K. L. (1978). Schooling and socioeconomic attainments: High school and college influences. *American Journal of Sociology, 84,* 319–347.
Gutteridge, T. G. (1971). *Career patterns of graduate business school alumni: An exploratory model.* Unpublished doctoral dissertation, Purdue University, West Lafayette, IN.
Haber, L. D., & McNeil, J. (1983). *Methodological questions in the estimation of disability prevalence.* Unpublished manuscript, Bureau of the Census, Population Division, Washington, DC.
Harlow, M. J. P., Fisher, S. D., & Monroe, D. F. (1974). *Postsecondary programs for the deaf: Follow-up data analysis.* (Monograph No. 5; report of USOE/BEH Grant No. OE-09-332189-4533-032). St. Paul: University of Minnesota, Center for Handicapped Children.
Hauser, R. M., & Featherman, D. L. (1977). *The process of stratification: Trends and analyses.* New York: Academic Press.
Hays, W. L. (1973). *Statistics for the social sciences* (2nd ed.). New York: Holt, Rinehart & Winston.
Henderson, M. T. (1966). Adult education—the beginning. *Proceedings of the Forty-second Meeting of the Convention of American Instructors of the Deaf.* Washington, DC: Government Printing Office.
Higgins, P. C. (1980). *Outsiders in a hearing world.* Beverly Hills, CA: Sage Publications.
Hodge, R. W., Seigel, P. M., & Rossi, P. H. (1966). Occupational prestige in the United States, 1925–1963. In R. Bendix & S. M. Lipset (Eds.), *Class, status and power.* New York: Free Press.
Indiana Jr. NAD Chapter. (n.d.). *Junior National Association of the Deaf.* Indianapolis: Author.

International Parents' Organization minutes. (1964). *Volta Review, 66,* 570.
Jarvik, L. F., Salzberger, R. M., & Falek, A. (1963). Deaf persons of outstanding achievement. In J. D. Rainer, K. Z. Altshuler, & F. J. Kallman (Eds.), *Family and mental health problems in a deaf population* (pp. 131–140). New York: Columbia University Press.
Jencks, C., Smith, M., Acland, H., Bane, M. J., Cohen, D., Gintis, H., Heyns, B., & Michelson, S. (1972). *Inequality: A reassessment of effects of family and schooling in America.* New York: Basic Books.
Jencks, C., Bartlett, S., Corcoran, M., Crouse, J., Eaglesfield, D., Jackson, G., McClelland, K., Mueser, P., Olneck, M., Schwartz, J., Ward, S., Williams, J. (1975). *Who gets ahead? The determinants of economic success in America.* New York: Basic Books.
Jensema, C. J., Karchmer, M. A., & Trybus, R. J. (1978). *The rated speech intelligibility of hearing-impaired children: Basic relationships and a detailed analysis* (Series R, No. 6). Washington, DC: Gallaudet College, Office of Demographic Studies.
Joiner, L. M., Erickson, E. L., & Crittenden, J. R. (1968). Occupational plans and aspirations of deaf adolescents. *Journal of Rehabilitation of the Deaf, 2*(3), 20–26.
Jordan, I. K., Gustason, G., & Rosen, R. (1974). An update on communication trends at programs for the deaf. *American Annals of the Deaf, 124,* 350–357.
Karchmer, M. A., Milone, M. N., Jr., & Wolk, S. (1979). Educational significance of hearing loss at three levels of severity. *American Annals of the Deaf, 124,* 97–109.
Katz, L. (n.d.). *IAPD: First report to the membership for the period of August 1971–December 1971.* Silver Spring, MD: International Association of Parents of the Deaf.
Kolvitz, M., & Ouellette, S. (1980). A comparison of sex-role attitudes of hearing and hearing-impaired young men. *Journal of Rehabilitation of the Deaf, 13*(4), 23–26.
Kolvolchuk, L. W., & Egelston, J. C. (1976). *Sex stereotyping of occupations by deaf and hearing adolescents.* Paper presented at the annual meeting of the American Personnel and Guidance Association, Chicago.

Kundert, J. J. (1969). Media services and captioned films. *Journal of Rehabilitation of the Deaf Monograph*, 2(5, Serial No. 1), 125–128.
Langlois, S. (1977). Les reseaux personnels et la diffusion des information sur des emplois. *Recherches Sociographiques*, 213–245.
Lauritsen, R. (1969). Report of the acting president. Proceedings of the second biennial convention, Professional Rehabilitation Workers with the Adult Deaf, Hot Springs, Arkansas, May 18–21, 1969. *Journal of Rehabilitation of the Deaf*, 2(1), 126–127.
Lerman, A. M., & Guilfoyle, G. R. (1970). *The development of prevocational behavior in deaf adolescents.* New York: Teachers College Press.
Lester, R. A. (1954). *Hiring practices and labor competition.* Princeton: Industrial Relation Section Report No. 88.
Lin, N., Ensel, W. M., & Vaughn, J. C. (1981). Social resources and strength of ties: Structural factors in occupational status attainment. *American Sociological Review*, 46, 393–405.
Lunde, A. S., & Bigman, S. K. (1959). *Occupational conditions among the deaf* (Final report of the Office of Vocational Rehabilitation Grant RD-79). Washington, DC: Gallaudet College and National Association of the Deaf (NARIC No. AN 79-03-X0048-1033).
Lurie, M., & Rayack, E. (1968). Racial differences in migration and job search: A case study. In L. Ferman, J. Kornbluth, & J. Miller (Eds.), *Negroes and jobs* (pp. 358–382). Ann Arbor: University of Michigan Press.
Markowicz, H., & Woodward, J. (1978). Language and the maintenance of boundaries in the deaf community. *Communication and Cognition*, 11, 29–38.
Martin, K. M. (1982, September). *Applied research and innovative practices in the placement and employment of hearing impaired college graduates.* Paper presented at the Arkansas Research and Training Center on Deafness and Hearing Impairment, Little Rock, AR.
Maxfield, B. D. (1982). *Science, engineering, and humanities doctorates in the United States: 1981.* Washington, DC: National Academy Press.

McKersie, R., & Ullman, J. (1966, September). Success patterns of MBA graduates. *Harvard Business School Bulletin*, 15–18.

Mead, G. H. (1964). *On social psychology.* Chicago: University of Chicago Press.

Meadow, K. P. (1967). The effect of early manual communication and family climate upon the deaf child's development (Doctoral dissertation, University of California, Berkeley; University Microfilms No. 68–5785).

Meek, P. G. (1968). The council concept. In H.G. Kopp (Ed.), *Accent on unity—Horizons of deafness: Social, communication, economic: Proceedings of National Forum, Council of Organizations Serving the Deaf* (pp. 19–23). Washington, DC: COSD.

Miller, D. C. (1970). *Handbook of research design and social measurement* (2nd ed.). New York: McKay.

Munson, H. L., & Miller, J. K. (1979). *Mainstreaming secondary level deaf students into occupational education* (Final Report of U.S. Office of Education Grant No. G007601433). Rochester, NY: University of Rochester.

Nash, J. E., & Nash, A. (1981). *Deafness in society.* Lexington, MA: DC Heath.

National Registry of Interpreters for the Deaf. (1979). *Deaf awareness.* Washington, DC: Author.

Nazzaro, J. N. (1977). *Exceptional timetables: Historic events affecting the handicapped and gifted.* Reston, VA: Council for Exceptional Children.

Norris, A. G. (Ed.). (1972). *Deafness: Contributed papers and reports of research and professional training programs on deafness* (Vol. 2) (SRS Final Report 22–P-55339/4–01). Silver Spring, MD: Professional Rehabilitation Workers with the Adult Deaf.

Oral Deaf Adults Section meeting. (1964). *Volta Review, 66,* 568–569.

Otto, L. B., & Haller, A. O. (1979). Evidence for a social psychological view of the status attainment process: Four studies compared. *Social Forces, 57*(3), 887–914.

Owens, J. A., Redden, M. R., & Brown, J. W. (1978). *Resource directory of handicaped scientists.* Washington, DC: American Association for the Advancement of Science.

Padden, C., & Markowicz, H. (1975). *Crossing cultural group boundaries into the deaf community*. Paper presented at the Conference on Culture and Communication, Temple University, Philadelphia.

Perrucci, C. (1978). Income attainment of college graduates: A comparison of employed men and women. *Sociology and Social Research, 62*, 361–386.

Perrucci, R., & Perrucci, C. (1970). Social origins, educational contexts, and career mobility. *American Sociological Review, 35*, 451–462.

Porter, J. N. (1974). Race, socialization, and mobility in educational and early occupational attainment. *American Sociological Review, 39*, 303–316.

Quigley, S. P., Jenne, W. C., & Phillips, S. B. (1968). *Deaf students in colleges and universities*. Washington, DC: A. G. Bell Association.

Rainer, J. D., Altshuler, K. Z., & Kallman, F. J. (1963). *Family and mental health problems in a deaf population*. New York: Columbia University Press.

Rawlings, B. W., & Jensema, C. J. (1977). *Two studies of the families of hearing impaired children* (Series R, No. 5, p. 5). Washington, DC: Gallaudet College.

Rawlings, B. W., Karchmer, M. A., & DeCaro, J. J. (1983). *College and career programs for deaf students, 1983 edition*. Washington, DC: Gallaudet College; Rochester, NY: National Technical Institute for the Deaf.

Rees, A. (1966). Information networks in labor markets. *American Economic Review, 56*, 559–566.

Rees, A., & Schultz, G. (1970). *Workers and wages in an urban labor market*. Chicago: University of Chicago Press.

Reid, G. L. (1972). Job search and the effectiveness of job-finding methods. *Industrial and Labor Relations Review, 25*, 479.

Reissman, L. (1959). *Class in American society*. New York: Free Press.

Rogers, E. M., & Kincaid, D. L. (1981). *Communication networks: Toward a new paradigm for research*. New York: Free Press.

Rogoff, N. (1953). Recent trends in urban occupational mobility. In R. Bendix & S. M. Lipset (Eds.), *Class, status, and power* (1st. ed.). New York: Free Press.

Rosenberg, S. M. (1981, Winter). Male occupational standing in the dual labor market. *Industrial Relations, 19*(1), 34–49.
Schein, J. D., & Delk, M. T., Jr. (1974). *The deaf population of the United States.* Silver Spring, MD: National Association of the Deaf.
Schein, J. D., Gentile, A., & Haase, K. W. (1970). *Development and evaluation of an expanded hearing loss scale questionnaire.* Washington, DC: U.S. Public Health Service Publication No. 1000 (Series 2, No. 37).
Schroedel, J. G. (1976/1977). Variables related to the attainment of occupational status among deaf adults. *Dissertation Abstracts International, 38*(2), 1048. (University Microfilms. No. 77–16, 447)
Schroedel, J. G. (1982a). *Socioeconomic attainment of technical college graduates who are deaf.* Paper presented at the annual Research Institute of the District of Columbia Sociological Society, Washington, DC.
Schroedel, J. G. (1982b). Surveys on the socioeconomic status of deaf adults, 1956–1981: Assessing response rates. In J. B. Christiansen & J. Egelston-Dodd (Eds.), *Socioeconomc status of the deaf population (Vol. 4).* Washington, DC: Gallaudet College.
Schroedel, J. G. (1984). Analyzing surveys of deaf adults: Implications for survey research on persons with disabilities. *Social Science Medicine, 19*, 619–627.
Schroedel, J. G. (1985). *The rehabilitation counselor and the hearing-impaired class of 1984 in postsecondary training programs.* Paper presented at the convention of the American Deafness and Rehabilitation Association, Little Rock, AR.
Schroedel, J. G., & Jacobsen, R. J. (1978). *Employer attitudes towards hiring persons with disabilities: A labor market research model.* Albertson, NY: Human Resources Center, Research Program Development Institute.
Schultz, G. P. (1962). A nonunion market for white-collar labor. In National Bureau of Economic Research, *Aspects of labor economics* (pp. 107–146). Princeton, NJ: Princeton University Press.
Sewell, W. H., Hauser, R. M., & Wolf, W. C. (1980). Sex, schooling, and occupational status. *American Journal of Sociology, 86*, 551–583.

Shapero, A. R., Howell, R., & Tombaugh, J. (1965). *The structure and dynamics of the defense R. and D. industry: The Los Angeles and Boston complexes.* Menlo Park, CA: Stanford Research Institute.
Shaposka, B. (1972). *The NAD story: A history of enlightened self-interest.* Silver Spring, MD: National Association of the Deaf.
Sheppard, H. L., & Belitsky, A. H. (1966). *The job hunt: Job seeking behavior of unemployed workers in a local economy.* Baltimore: Johns Hopkins University Press.
Sjoberg, G. (1960). *The preindustrial city.* New York: Free Press.
Spaeth, J. L. (1977). Differences in the occupational achievement process between male and female college graduates. *Sociology of Education, 50,* 206–217.
Spitze, G., & Spaeth, J. L. (1977). *Human capital investments of married female college graduates* (Working papers in Applied Social Statistics WP7703). Urbana: University of Illinois, Department of Sociology.
Spragins, A. B., Karchmer, M. A., & Schildroth, A. N. (1981). Profile of psychological service providers to hearing-impaired students. *American Annals of the Deaf, 126,* 94–105.
Stokoe, W. C., Jr., Croneberg, C. G., & Casterline, D. (1965). *A dictionary of American Sign Language on linguistics principles.* Washington, DC: Gallaudet College Press.
Strassler, B. (1982). *1983 international telephone directory of the deaf.* Silver Spring, MD: Telecommunications for the Deaf, Inc.
Stumpf, S. A., & Colarelli, S. M. (1980). Career exploration: Development dimensions and some preliminary findings. *Psychological Reports, 47,* 979–988.
Super, D. E. (1957). *The psychology of careers.* New York: Harper & Row.
Theodorson, G. A., & Theodorson, A. G. (1969). *Modern dictionary of sociology.* New York: Crowell.
Tolbert C. M, II. (1982). Industrial segmentation and men's career mobility. *American Sociological Review, 47,* 457–477.
Trusheim, D., & Crouse, J. (1980). *Effects of college prestige on men's occupational status and earnings.* Paper presented at the annual meeting of the American Educational Research Association, Boston.

Trusheim, D., & Crouse, J. (1981). Effects of college prestige on men's occupational status and income. *Research in Higher Education, 14*(4), 283-304.

Ullman, J. C., & Taylor, D. P. (1965). The information system in changing labor markets. In G. G. Somers (Ed.), *Proceedings of the Industrial Relations Research Association* (276-289). Madison, WI: IRRA.

United States Senate. (1973). *Vocational rehabilitation* (Report No. 93-391). Washington, DC: Government Printing Office.

U.S. General Accounting Office (1985). *Educating students at Gallaudet and the National Technical Institute for the Deaf: Who are served and what are the costs?* Washington, DC: Government Printing Office. [GAO/HRD 85-34]

Walker, B. L. (1982). The relationship between teacher expectations and the occupational aspirations of seniors in selected residential schools for the deaf. *Directions, 2*(4), 35-44.

Walter, V. (Ed.). (1982, October 25). EPOC helps students get off-campus work experience. *On the Green*, 1. (Available from Gallaudet University, Washington, DC 20002)

Wax, T. M., & Danek, M. M. (1982). Deaf women and double jeopardy: Challenge for research and practice. In A. Boros & R. Stuckless (Eds.), *Deaf people and social change* (Vol. 4, pp. 177-196). Washington, DC: Gallaudet College.

Wells, D. O. (1969). The Delgado College academic and vocational education program for the deaf. *Journal of Rehabilitation of the Deaf, 3*, 44-51.

Welniak, E. J., & Henson, M. F. (1984). *Money income of households, families, and persons in the United States: 1982* (Current Population Reports, Series P-60, No. 142). Washington, DC: Bureau of the Census.

Youngs, J., Jr. (1967). Interpreting for deaf clients. *Journal of Rehabilitation of the Deaf, 1*, 49.

Index

Academic preparation, 16–18. *See also* Education; Educational attainment
Accommodation, in employment, 172–174
Acoustic coupler, 5
Actors, 9, 26
Administrative personnel, 26
Age at onset of hearing impairment. *See* Communication, and age at onset of hearing impairment; Educational attainment, and age at onset of hearing impairment; Hearing impairment, age at onset of; Occupational status, and age at onset of hearing impairment; Speech skills, and age at onset of hearing impairment
Age of occurrence of hearing impairment. *See* Age at onset of hearing impairment
Alexander G. Bell Association for the Deaf (AGBAD), 5, 21
Allen, R. E., 49–50

American Deafness and Rehabilitation Association (ADARA), 6, 21
American Sign Language (ASL), 6, 7. *See also* Communication modes, sign language
American Society for Deaf Children (ASDC), 7
Attitudes. *See also* Deaf awareness
  employers', 167, 169–170, 174–175
  hearing-impaired workers', 180
Audiometers, 191
Audiometry, 192
Automation, 167, 168

Babbidge report, 6
Bell scholarships, 8
Blue-collar workers. *See* Workers, blue-collar
Bureau of Education of the Handicapped, 7

CAID (Convention of American Instructors of the Deaf), 21

California State University, Northridge (CSUN), 4, 42, 148, 169, 186
Captioned films for the deaf, 3, 6
Captioned television, 9
CEASD (Conference of Educational Administrators Serving the Deaf), 21
Certification of teachers. *See* Teachers, certification of
Civil rights. *See* Legal rights
Colleges
  general, 148
  type of, 113–114
Communication, 20, 21, 25–33, 177
  and age at onset of hearing impairment, 142–145
  aids to, 163
  barriers to, 31
  with co-workers, 140, 141
  educators' philosophy of, 102
  interpreters role in, 163
  parental inadequacy in, 95, 96
  preferred method of, 63, 64
  social, 28
  telecommunication devices for, 163
  total communication, 63, 64
  at work, 27, 28, 144, 173
Communication modes
  fingerspelling, 26, 27, 140
  manual, 26, 32, 103, 140, 141, 182
  non-oral, 142, 143
  oral, 26, 28, 103, 140–144, 177, 184
  sign language, 25–28, 32, 63, 64, 81, 101, 140, 162, 177, 191
  speech, 25–28, 32, 63, 64, 101, 141, 142, 162, 191
  speechreading, 26–30, 32, 63, 64, 140, 141, 143, 144, 157, 177, 191
  use of, in labor market sectors, 81
  writing, 26, 27, 63, 64, 140, 141, 191
Communication Skills Program, 7, 141
Community organizations, participation in, 22, 23
Continuing education, 4
Council of Organizations Serving the Deaf (COSD), 7

Counselors. *See* Rehabilitation services
Coye, Terry H., 47
Crammatte, Alan B., 51, 52, 93, 95, 101, 105, 126, 130, 133, 136, 139, 148

Day classes, 36, 37. *See also* Schools, public, with program for hearing-impaired students
Deaf awareness, ix, 7, 9, 171, 175, 180–182
Deaf community, 50, 62, 148, 180, 188
Deafness. *See also* Hearing impairment, definitions of, extent of
  adventitious, 142, 145
Deafness Research and Training Center, New York University, 6, 10
Deaf sector, 80–83, 130, 140, 149, 165, 177, 181, 182, 184, 189. *See also* Job finding methods, deaf sector
  communication in, 81, 177
  definition of, 60, 74, 189
  employees' aspirations, 90–91
  employers, 74
  job categories, 77–79
  job satisfaction in, 84–85
  perceived rejection in, 86–88
Decibels (dB), as measure of hearing loss, 191–194
Delgado Community College, 8
Dictionary of American Sign Language, 6
Discrimination. *See* Rejection
Dream jobs, 90, 91
Duncan, O. D., 15, 90, 107
Duncan scale. *See* Socioeconomic index (SEI)

Education, 35–46, 167
  areas of concentration in, 40–42, 118
  attitudes of youth, 118
  and college type, 99, 100
  expectations of parents, 98, 99

expectations of teachers, 98–101
and gender, 118, 121–122
higher, 147, 148, 180
least restrictive environment, 10
role of, in employment, 168, 169
and school type, 99, 100
support services in, 39–41, 136, 147
Educational aspirations, 96–99, 120
and college type, 106
and school type, 106
Educational attainment, 17, 18, 37, 38–39, 44, 93, 96, 97, 106, 128, 129, 136, 177, 178
and age, 104, 105, 114, 115, 133, 137, 179
and age at onset of hearing impairment, 38, 39, 101, 102, 104, 105, 110, 111, 113, 115, 133, 135, 137, 146, 179
and college type, 106, 107, 110, 113, 133, 135, 137, 148, 149
and communication, 102
comparisons of, 146, 179, 181
difficulties in, 39, 146, 147
and extent of hearing impairment, 37, 110–113, 115, 133
and gender, 98, 101, 118, 121, 122
and occupational status, 116–117
and parental status, 102, 104, 105, 150, 151
of parents, 94, 95, 103
and parents' occupations, 101
predictors of, 115, 116
and race, 98
and reading ability, 102
of respondents vs. general population, 43
and salaries, 44, 45, 152, 153
and school type, 98, 99, 101–107, 110, 147–149
and sign language, 102
and socioeconomic status, 145
and speech skills, 39, 40, 102–107, 133, 135, 137, 179
Educational settings. *See* Schools
Education for All Handicapped Children Act. *See* Public Law 94-142

Employers
attitudes of, 167, 169–170, 181
educational institutions, 19, 26, 67, 68, 70, 73, 74, 77
government agencies, 19, 26, 67, 68, 74, 77
hospitals, 19, 74
and preferred method of communication, 68
private business, 19, 26, 67, 68, 70, 74, 77
religious organizations, 19, 74
Employment
accommodation in, 172, 173
administrative positions in, 181
automation in, 167–168
barriers, 35, 69
blue-collar vs. white-collar, 168
career ladders, 174
as educators, 1960 vs. 1982, 180
expanding opportunities in, 181
legal rights in, 170, 171, 180
of 1960 vs. 1982 respondents, 183, 184
paternalism in, 174
perspectives, 167–175
qualifications needed for, 171
self-, 19, 26
seminars, 11
summer, 172
Experiential Programs Off Campus (EPOC), 10, 171

Fingerspelling. *See* Communication modes, fingerspelling
Fort Monroe workshops, 2, 3

Gallaudet College, x, 3, 10, 101, 148, 168–169
age of students at, 41
alumni 6, 148, 187
socioeconomic attainment of, 127
survey respondents, 41
Centennial Fund, 5, 8
Experiential Programs Off Campus (EPOC), 10, 171–172
Graduate Fellowship Fund, 5, 8
job placement program, 171–172

Gallaudet College (*continued*)
  role of gender in selecting majors at, 118
  social work major, 75
Gallaudet University. *See* Gallaudet College
Granovetter, Mark S., 48–49, 51, 56–58

Halex House, 9
Hearing Ability Scale, 191–194
Hearing aids, 140, 163
Hearing impaired, x, 188. *See also* Hearing impairment
Hearing impairment. *See also* Educational attainment, and age at onset of hearing impairment
  age of onset of, 30, 31, 37–39, 103, 144, 177
  definitions of, x, 188
  extent of, 140, 153, 179, 191–193
  impact of, on speech skills, 29–31
  and job sector choice, 80–81
  in 1982 respondents, 193–194
  and type of college attended, 113
  and type of high school attended, 36–37
  of 1960 vs. 1982 respondents, 155
Hearing sector, 21–22, 80–83. *See also* Job finding methods, hearing sector
  communication in, 81, 177, 182
  comparison of 1960 vs. 1982 respondents in, 139–166, 179–180, 184
  definition of, 60, 74, 189
  employees' aspirations, 90–91
  employers, 74
  job categories, 77–79
  job satisfaction in, 84–85
  perceived rejection in, 86, 88–89
Higgins, P. C., 50

IAPD (International Association of Parents of the Deaf), 7
IBM Corporation (International Business Machine Corporation), 10, 172, 185
Income, psychic, 19. *See also* Salaries

Independence, 174–175
Interdependence, 175
Internships, 171–172
Interpreters/Interpreting. *See also* Communication, interpreters
  role in
  RID (Registry of Interpreters for the Deaf), 5
  for students, 40, 136
  in workplace, 140, 163, 173, 182
IPO (International Parents Organization), 5

Jamison, Steven L., 167, 181, 185
Jencks, C., 13, 16, 150
Job finding methods, 47, 56
  in deaf sector, 64–66, 69, 178
  definition of, 53, 189
  direct application, 48, 49, 54, 55, 57, 58, 60–69, 189
  formal means, 48, 49, 54, 55, 57, 58, 60, 61, 64–69, 178
  in hearing sector, 64–66, 69, 178
  informal means, 48, 49
  and job satisfaction, 58
  and labor market sectors, 60, 61, 64–67, 69
  networks, 48–51, 59, 60–67, 70, 182
  personal contacts, 48, 49, 53–55, 57, 58, 60–62, 64, 65, 68, 69, 178, 189
  and preferred methods of communication, 64, 65, 68, 69
  of professional, technical, and managerial workers, 48
  and salaries, 57
Job satisfaction, 20, 73, 75–77, 165, 178–179, 213–214. *See also* Labor market sectors, job satisfaction
  of 1960 vs. 1982 respondents, 165, 180
Junior National Association of the Deaf (JRNAD), 3

Keaveny, T. J., 49–50
Kellogg Foundation, 11
Kendall Demonstration Elementary School for the Deaf (KDES), 9

Labor market sectors, 73–74. *See also* Communication modes, use of, in labor market sectors; Deaf sector; Hearing sector
  comparison of supervisory duties, 83–84
  division by gender, 75
  extent of hearing impairment in, 80–81
  influence of school type, 81–82
  job satisfaction in, 84–85
  occupational categories, 77–79
  perceived rejection in, 86–89
  promotions in, 83
  salary comparison, 82–83
Labor market studies, 47
Language acquisition, 31, 143
Leadership Training Program in the Area of Deafness (LTP), 4
Legal Defense Fund (of NAD), 11
Legal rights, 10, 182. *See also* Employment, legal rights
Linguistics, 31
Lipreading. *See* Communication modes, speechreading

Mental health services, 3
Merit awards, 164
Methodology
  for calculating job satisfaction and rejection indexes, 213–214
  canvass of 1960 and 1982 respondents, 185–187
  for compiling 1982 mailing list, 185–187
  confidentiality of, 187
  in Coye's study, 51–53
  in Crammatte's study, 183–190
  criteria for selection, 139, 140, 185
  for measuring extent and age at onset of hearing impairment, 191–194
  of questionnaire, 185, 187, 188
  response rate, 187
  in Schroedel's study, 107–110
Mobility
  demand, 125
  and education, 95
  of hearing impaired vs. hearing workers, 95
  occupational, 93, 96, 106, 132, 179, 182
  and gender, 122–125
  social, 16
  social-distance, 125
  socioeconomic, 184
Model Secondary School for the Deaf (MSSD), 6
Multiple regression, 179
  limitation for present data, 109, 110

National Association of the Deaf (NAD), 4, 5, 9, 10, 141
  Communication Skills Program, 7
  executive secretary, 7
  Legal Defense Fund, 11
National Census of the Deaf Population (NCDP), 15–17, 38, 126
National Center for Law and the Deaf (NCLD), 10–11
National Center on Employment of the Deaf (at NTID), 11, 172
National Technical Institute for the Deaf (NTID), 8, 120, 148, 169
  occupational status of graduates, 17, 126, 127, 130, 132
  regional employment seminars, 11
  role of gender in selecting majors at, 118
  social service majors at, 75
  support services, 39–40
  survey respondents from, 41–42, 185, 187
National Theatre of the Deaf (NTD), 7, 9
Networks, of deaf people, 50. *See also* Job finding methods, networks
New York State Psychiatric Institute, 3

Occupational aspirations, 95–98, 100
  parental influence on, 120–121
  and school type, 106–107
Occupational categories, 14, 15, 78, 79, 154, 160
Occupational expectations, 121
Occupational mobility. *See* Mobility, occupational
Occupational status, 50, 96–99, 128–129, 177, 182

Occupational status (*continued*)
    and age, 104, 105
    and age at onset of hearing impairment, 101, 105–107, 179
    and college type, 106, 107, 136
    and educational attainment, 38, 104–109, 116–117, 126, 127, 134–136, 138, 179
    and extent of hearing impairment, 179
    and gender, 101, 107, 118–123, 125–126, 127, 129, 131, 134–136
    of hearing-impaired workers, 102, 103
    of hearing vs. hearing-impaired workers, 126–132
    influence of parental status on, 14, 94–96, 101, 103–105, 116, 122–126, 134–136, 138, 179
    predictors of, 116–126
    research on, 93, 105–107
    social psychological model, 96–101
    socioeconomic attainments, 101–105
    socioeconomic status, 94–96
    and school type, 101
    and speech skills, 104, 105, 107
    stereotypes, 119, 134, 182
Occupations, 190, 205–212. *See also* Occupational status, influence of parental status on
    and age at onset of hearing impairment, 156
    blue-collar, 155
    Bureau of the Census classifications of, 14, 15
    career learning of, 120
    categories of, 154, 155
    counseling, 120
    and economic conditions, 152–161
    and gender, 118–120
    gender stereotypes of, 120
    of general population, 15
    high status, 130–132, 136
    of 1960 vs. 1982 respondents, 154, 155
    of parents, 15
    pink-collar, 155
    professional, 188
    professional, technical, and managerial, 19, 77–79
    of respondents, 18, 19, 205–212
    white-collar, 155
    of women, 155
Office of Vocational Rehabilitation (OVR), 3
On-the-job-training, 173
Oral Deaf Adults Section (ODAS), Alexander Graham Bell Association for the Deaf, 5, 186

Paternalism, 148
    in employment, 174
Predictors of educational and occupational attainment, 98, 102, 103, 105, 109, 110, 114–117, 129, 136
Professional affiliations, 21–22
Professional Rehabilitation Workers with the Adult Deaf (PRWAD). *See* American Deafness and Rehabilitation Association
Promotions, 20, 164, 165. *See also* Labor market sectors, promotions
Psychological service workers, 26
Public Law 87-276, 4
Public Law 91-587, 9
Public Law 94-142 (Education for All Handicapped Children Act), 10, 181

Registry of Interpreters for the Deaf (RID), 5, 21
Regression analysis, 137
Rehabilitation Act. *See* Vocational Rehabilitation Act of 1973
Rehabilitation counselors. *See* Rehabilitation services
Rehabilitation services, 26, 32, 55, 174
Rejection, 13, 14, 20, 21, 70, 164. *See also* Hearing sector, perceived rejection in
    in deaf sector, 86–88
    at educational institutions, 86–88

in hearing sector, 25, 86, 88–89
indexes of 21, 216
Riverside Community College, 4

St. Paul Technical/Vocational Institute (TVI), 8
Salaries, 19, 152, 165, 184. *See also* Labor market sectors, salary comparison
  and age, 158
  and communication modes, 159, 161
  in deaf sector, 77, 179
  of deaf women, 76–77
  and educational attainment, 44–45, 151–152, 180
  by gender, 76, 159
  in hearing sector, 77, 179
  of 1960 vs. 1982 respondents, 151, 152, 157, 158, 180
  and occupations, 159, 160
  and speech skills, 158, 162
Schools
  counseling offices in, 26
  day, 37, 99, 147, 184
  general (public), 36, 37, 82, 147
  hearing-impaired teachers in, 79, 80, 148
  with program for hearing-impaired students, 36, 37, 147, 184
  residential, 35–37, 99, 100, 121, 147, 181, 184
  special programs in, 82
Schroedel, John G., 16–17, 38, 95, 102–103, 105, 142–143
Seattle Community College, 8
Self-concept, 96
Sign language. *See* Communication modes, sign language
Social psychological model, 93, 96–101, 120
Social workers, 26, 32
Socioeconomic achievements of deaf people, 93
Socioeconomic attainments, 101–105. *See also* Mobility; Occupational status
Socioeconomic equality, 125, 129, 136

Socioeconomic Index (SEI) scores, 15, 107–109, 130–132, 133–134
  of deaf women's jobs, 121, 127, 129–130, 132
  of dream jobs, 90–91
  of hearing vs. hearing-impaired college alumni, 126–127, 129–130, 136
  of respondents and their parents, 123–126
  of respondents' jobs, 116–117
Socioeconomic status, 13, 35. *See also* Occupational status
  and educational attainment, 145
  hypothetical variable of, 13–16
  parental, 13–16, 93, 94–96, 98, 100, 101, 103, 106, 179
  and status of occupations, 108
  of women, 127
Southwest Collegiate Institute for the Deaf (SWCID), 11, 196
Special School of the Future Project, 11
Speech. *See* Communication modes, speech
Speechreading. *See* Communication modes, speechreading
Speech skills, 27–29, 103, 141–143, 162, 177
  and age at onset of hearing impairment, 30–31, 112, 143–145
  and college type, 114
  and educational attainment, 39–40, 103, 179
  and extent of hearing impairment, 29–30, 112

Teachers. *See also* Schools, general, hearing-impaired teachers in
  certification of, 37–38, 148
  in deaf sector, 86–88, 178, 181
  in hearing sector, 148
  job satisfaction of, 20, 165
  in 1960 study, 149
  upward mobility of, 149–150
  use of sign language by, 25–26, 32
TDD. *See* Telecommunication devices for the deaf (TDD)

Technicians, 153, 155
Telecommunication Devices for the Deaf (TDD), 5, 8, 163, 173, 182. *See also* Communication, telecommunication devices for the deaf
Telecommunications for the Deaf, Inc. (TDI), 8
Total communication (TC), 8, 63, 64

Vocational Rehabilitation Act of 1973, 9, 10, 40, 148, 170

Weitbrecht, Robert, 5
White-collar families, 150
White-collar workers. *See* Workers, white-collar
Williams, Boyce R., 3
Workers
  blue-collar, 15, 48
  families of, 150
  older, 189
  pink-collar, 155
  professional, technical, and managerial, 17, 48
  white-collar, 15, 48
  younger, 189
Working conditions, 73–92
Writing. *See* Communication modes, writing